Feeding the preterm infant

A practical handbook

Dr. Fook-Choe Cheah

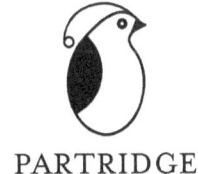

PARTRIDGE

Copyright © 2017 by Fook-Choe Cheah.

Library of Congress Control Number: 2016962096
ISBN: Hardcover 978-1-4828-8166-0
Softcover 978-1-4828-8165-3
eBook 978-1-4828-8167-7

All rights reserved. No part of this book may be used or reproduced by any means, graphic, electronic, or mechanical, including photocopying, recording, taping or by any information storage retrieval system without the written permission of the author except in the case of brief quotations embodied in critical articles and reviews.

Because of the dynamic nature of the Internet, any web addresses or links contained in this book may have changed since publication and may no longer be valid. The views expressed in this work are solely those of the author and do not necessarily reflect the views of the publisher, and the publisher hereby disclaims any responsibility for them.

Print information available on the last page.

To order additional copies of this book, contact
Toll Free 800 101 2657 (Singapore)
Toll Free 1 800 81 7340 (Malaysia)
orders.singapore@partridgepublishing.com

www.partridgepublishing.com/singapore

Dedicated to

My Loving and Gracious Heavenly Father
who inspired me to part with this humble contribution to share in
enriching the lives of others.

The memory of my late father.

My loving mother
who is the best self-taught nutritionist, her untiring efforts
in reminding me of optimum nutrition for a healthy living
and enjoying the fruits of life harvests.

My precious patients and their parents
who have taught me all the finer complementary knowledge and
true insights in nutrition no books can teach in practice.

To my beloved pet beagle, whose constant staying awake
to faithfully greet me with her unconditional affection when I
leave for and return from work, makes a long day
so much more tenable.

Table of contents

	List of contributors	3
	Foreword	4
	List of abbreviations	5
	Introduction	6
Chapter 1	Parenteral nutrition as an integral component of nutritional support of the preterm infant	9
Chapter 2	Early enteral nutrition and feeding strategies for the preterm infant during the acute period of illness	21
Chapter 3	Strategies towards successful breastfeeding and individualising nutritional needs of the preterm infant	31
Chapter 4	Monitoring and optimising growth of stable preterm infants in the convalescent phase	45
Chapter 5	Strategies and challenges in feeding the preterm infant with intrauterine growth retardation	53
Chapter 6	Post-discharge feeding for long term growth and health	61
Chapter 7	Prebiotics and probiotics: relevance and impact on preterm nutrition (in the Asian context)	69
Chapter 8	Cultural beliefs and practices influencing breastfeeding of the preterm infant - *A survey of reported experiences from neonatologists in the Asian region*	81
Chapter 9	Illustrative case series with Q &A	89
	Appendices	121
	References	135

List of contributors

Fook-Choe Cheah
MD, MRCPI, MMed (Paediatrics), FRACP, FRCPCH, FAMM, PhD

Department Of Paediatrics,
Universiti Kebangsaan Malaysia Medical Centre,
Kuala Lumpur,
MALAYSIA

Girish Deshpande
FRACP, MSc

Department of Neonatal Paediatrics,
Nepean Hospital Sydney;
Sydney Medical School Nepean,
University of Sydney,
AUSTRALIA

Jiun Lee
MBBS, MMed

Department of Neonatology,
National University Hospital,
SINGAPORE

Le-Ye Lee
MBBS, MMed (Paediatrics), MRCPCH

Department of Neonatology,
National University Hospital,
SINGAPORE

Sanjay Patole
FRACP, DrPH

Department of Neonatal Paediatrics,
KEM Hospital for Women;
Western Australia Centre for Neonatal Research and Education,
University of Western Australia,
AUSTRALIA

Foreword

It is my great pleasure to write a foreword for the book, "Feeding the Preterm Infant", spearheaded by Prof. Dr. Cheah. There have been tremendous advances in the care of the premature infant over the last few decades, especially in the survival of even very small infants. Worldwide, there is little question that nutritional support of these premature infants has now become a major issue, in an attempt to protect and preserve the vital organs of the infant as a foundation for a healthy life.

This book will thus be extremely helpful to general paediatricians, neonatal specialty trainees, and medical nursing and dietetic students, putting into special perspective the social and cultural practices that affect infant nutrition, especially in the Asian world. It is important not only to understand the physiology of the growing premature infant, but also to put into practice effective ways of ensuring excellent nutrition in these infants, particularly in countries with varying resources, practices, and cultural concerns. Diseases such as necrotising enterocolitis have varying incidences in different parts of the world, and these present particularly challenging situations. Post-discharge feeding practices are variable, and particularly difficult in situations of disadvantaged nutritional nutrition and growth restriction, requiring special effort for effective catch up growth in these infants.

The book attempts to understand the impact of complex cultural beliefs and practices on nutrition issues such as breastfeeding in the premature infant. I particularly appreciate the use of case studies which illustrate actual nutritional practices in various settings, which will be helpful for practitioners to understand real-life situations.

There have been great advances since the first Vitamin and Mineral Requirements in Preterm Infant book that I edited in 1984, to our subsequent iterations of the classic Nutrition for the Preterm Infant books in 1993, 2005 and 2014. It is a privilege to see the practical impact of advancing nutrition knowledge on the actual care of our precious infants, especially in an Asian setting. I trust that you will use this book wisely and helpfully.

Reginald Tsang
Professor Emeritus of Pediatrics,
Cincinnati Children's Hospital, USA

List of abbreviations

AGA	Appropriate for gestational age	lcGOS	Long chain galacto-oligosaccharide
BPA	Bisphenol A	LCPUFAs	Long-chain polyunsaturated fatty acids
BUN	Blood urea nitrogen	LOS	Late onset sepsis
CI	Confidence interval	MCT	Medium chain triglyceride
CLD	Chronic lung disease	MDI	Mental development index
CMV	Human cytomegalovirus	MEF	Minimal enteral feeding
CONS	Coagulase-negative staphylococci	NDI	Neurodevelopmental impairment
CPAP	Continuous positive airway pressure	NEC	Necrotising enterocolitis
CRP	C-reactive protein	NICU	Neonatal intensive care unit
DHA	Docosahexaenoic acid	NP-CPAP	Nasal prong continuous positive airway pressure
DSLNT	Disialyllacto-N-tetraose	OR	Odds ratio
EBM	Expressed breast milk	OS	Oligosaccharides
ELBW	Extremely low birth weight	PCA	Post-conceptional age
ESPGHAN	European Society for Paediatric Gastroenterology, Hepatology and Nutrition	PDA	Patent ductus arteriosus
GER	Gastro-oesophageal reflux	PDF	Post-discharge formula
GH	Growth hormone	PDI	Psychomotor developmental index
GI	Gastrointestinal	PICC	Peripheral inserted central catheter
GIT	Gastrointestinal tract	RCT	Randomised controlled trial
GIR	Glucose infusion rate	RTF	Ready to feed
GRV	Gastric residual volume	scGOS	Short chain galacto-oligosaccharide
Hb A	Adult haemoglobin	SGA	Small for gestational age
Hb F	Foetal haemoglobin	SVC	Superior vena cava
HMF	Human milk fortifier	TG	Triglyceride
HMO	Human milk oligosaccharide	TFEF	Time to full enteral feeds
Ig A	Immunoglobulin A	TLR	Toll-like receptors
IGFBP	Insulin-like growth factor-binding protein	TPN	Total parenteral nutrition
IUGR	Intrauterine growth restriction	UKM	Universiti Kebangsaan Malaysia
IVH	Intraventricular haemorrhage	VLBW	Very low birth weight
KMC	Kangaroo mother care	WHO	World Health Organization
LBW	Low birth weight	WMD	Weighted mean difference
lcFOS	Long chain fructo-oligosaccharides		

Introduction

The World Health Organization (WHO) reports that annually an estimated 15 million babies are born preterm and this number is rising. Complications related to prematurity also contribute as a major cause of death in children under five years of age and about three quarters could be prevented with cost-effective interventions. Nutrition provided through breastfeeding supported by kangaroo mother care (KMC) nursing are two initiatives that could reduce mortality rates even in resource poor countries. It is thus timely and appropriate that I took up the task to produce a handbook that compiles the current evidence and practices in nutrition management of the preterm infant, particularly from a local and regional perspective. While this area is one of the most rapidly evolving in the science of nutrition, in most neonatal intensive care units (NICU) or nurseries, the art of handling this specialised niche is often led by neonatologists, who formulate the standard operating procedures often with great variability between localities. To dietitians and nutritionists, this field is rather sub-specialised and warrants specific training before they would consider engaging in it full-time. Furthermore, in many parts of Asia, a significant proportion of paediatric practice involves neonatology and a strong understanding of the nutritional needs of the preterm infant based on the current scientific evidence will contribute to improved outcomes. This region also happens to have one of the largest population of preterm births.

In this practical handbook, I have included a personal "flavour" of my own perspectives as a practising neonatologist into the potpourri of the fundamentals of nutrition management of the preterm infant. The topics selected cover core issues commonly encountered and include the extremely preterm who needs early parenteral nutrition support and minimal enteral feeding, the preterm intrauterine growth restricted/small for gestational age infants (IUGR/SGA) with feeding intolerance and a greater risk of necrotising enterocolitis (NEC), monitoring the adequacy in enteral nutrition that could modify outcomes of growth and development among stable, "awaiting to go home" infants, and optimal nutrition continuation post-hospital discharge. The ethnic diversity and unique multi-cultural environment in the Asian region and the potential impact that this may have on feeding the preterm infant has inspired the inclusion of a chapter that explores various common issues encountered by practitioners here. It is hoped that this may spur further collaborative research efforts to find solutions to the priority issues. This handbook is primarily for the readership of paediatricians, neonatal and paediatric fellow in training, medical students, as well as advanced nursing and dietetic students. In order to make it a truly practical handbook that could be used as an introductory and mid-level resource for teaching and training purposes, the final chapter discusses ten instructive case studies illustrating some of the commonly managed feeding problems in the preterm infant. The appendix also contains important reference ranges of nutrient composition of breast milk, milk substitutes and fortifiers, and adapted feeding protocols.

Finally, this book would not have been completed if not for the contributions from key people that I am most grateful to. I am honoured to have Professor Emeritus Dr. Reginald Tsang, whose book "Nutrition of the Preterm Infant" has been one of the core references for neonatologists, writing the foreword. He also advised the inclusion of "a lot of case studies" for a handbook to be a practical one, which I agreed and followed whole-heartedly. I am also grateful for my colleagues in Singapore and Australia who contributed in authoring several key chapters and case studies; Dr. Lee Le Ye and Associate Professor Lee Jiun, are also my collaborators in studying growth outcomes in preterm infants in Singapore and Malaysia. Dr. Deshpande and Professor Patole, whose vast expertise and experience in examining probiotics use, with their discourse provide a valuable and essential resource in evaluating the logistics and potential future introduction of this therapy in this region. Also to my junior faculty members, Drs. Joyce Hong and Wan Nurulhuda, and fellow-in-training, Dr. Eunice Tiew, I accord my sincere gratitude for their effort in compiling the case studies that we managed together in the NICU of the University Kebangsaan Malaysia Medical Centre (UKMMC). Last but not least, I wish to thank my good friend and colleague, Professor of Early Life Nutrition, University of Amsterdam, Dr. Ruurd Van Elburg, for his critique and comments during the production of this book. My appreciation and gratitude also goes out to Mediconnexions Consulting Sdn Bhd for providing the editorial support.

Dr. Fook-Choe Cheah
Professor of Paediatrics (Neonatology)
Universiti Kebangsaan Malaysia Medical Centre
Kuala Lumpur, Malaysia

Chapter 1

Parenteral nutrition as an integral component of nutritional support of the preterm infant

- Fook-Choe Cheah -

What is known on this topic?

- Total parenteral nutrition (TPN) is crucial before enteral feeding can be established.
- Aggressive advancement of TPN is also effective and safe but keeping infants on TPN for a prolonged period can be risky.
- For preterm infants, especially those with very low birth weight (VLBW), TPN should be started within the first 24 hours of life.
- At least 1.5 g/kg/day protein should be provided from Day 1 to avoid catabolism.

What this chapter adds?

- Practical tips and information on how to set up basic TPN support in resource limited centres.
- Basic non-compounded TPN can be prepared by most neonatal units using a simple and practical formula.
- TPN should be utilised for the shortest duration possible (typically not more than 10–14 days) to avert the risk of catheter related sepsis and cholestasis.
- TPN should be regarded as a crucial interim "bridging-the-gap" while awaiting enteral feeding to be fully established.
- Summary, practical tips and links to resources useful as guides for intravenous line access placement.

Introduction

The limited nutrient stores in low birth weight (LBW) preterm infants with the relatively high energy expended not only for thermoregulation, but also in overcoming illnesses, increase their risk of spiralling into a catabolic state. Gut immaturity and a delay in establishing enteral feeds further complicates this potentially rapid developing catabolic state, equating this to a "nutritional emergency" that needs urgent attention and intervention. TPN is the vital "bridging-the-gap" approach, and it is important that every neonatal intensive care unit (NICU) caring for high risk preterm infants recognise the importance of this essential component of nutritional support. Most resource limited units should be able to provide some basic form of non-compounded TPN in the interim period. Pharmacy support in compounding or administering TPN services, available in many other centres however, ensures sterile TPN therapy in the longer term.

The preterm infant's gut and feeding intolerance

The gastrointestinal tract (GIT) is formed by 10 weeks of gestation. Within 20 weeks of gestation, intrinsic factors such as glycoprotein important for vitamin B_{12} absorption, pepsin, and enzymes that digest lactose and other carbohydrate are present. Although GI motor activity can be detected by the 24th week, organised peristalsis is only established within 29–30 weeks.[1]

Some aspects of the growth and maturation of the GI tract are determined by the specific gestational age,[2] while others can be affected by nutrition.[3] In the preterm infant, the immature gut lacks the capability for nutrient absorption and utilisation. In addition to the functional immaturity of the gut, premature infants have undeveloped mucosal barrier function and immune response, and greater risk of pathogenic bacterial colonisation. These factors lead to intestinal inflammation and injury, as well as necrotising enterocolitis (NEC). Nutrient deprivation is further aggravated by feeding intolerance, fluid restriction, concurrent illnesses, and energy for thermal balance. The particular groups at risk are the moderate to severe preterm infants (< 34 weeks) and VLBW infants (lower than 1500 g).

In the above context, parenteral nutrition is vital as a kick-start nutritional emergency intervention. Even so, minimal enteral feeds to prime the gut should be started concurrently within the first 24 hours of life. It has previously been thought that nutrition for infants can be deferred for the first 48 hours, but it has been shown that preterm infants fed with glucose alone in the early days after birth, experience a reduction in body protein compared to a foetus of the same gestation age who is developing in the womb (Figure 1).[4] Growth is about the balance between energy and protein intake, and optimal intakes of protein with energy can stop growth failure.[5] Extrauterine energy requirements of the preterm infant however do not equate foetal energy expenditures-accretion balance because of various external stresses comprising lower ambient temperatures, physical activity from breathing, and immune regulatory function to ward of infections in a hostile microbial environment. Extra energy requirements have to cater for these conditions in order that sufficient energy is spared for growth.

Figure 1. Change in body protein over the first 7 days of post-natal life for a 1000 g, 26 week gestation infant provided just glucose versus in utero.[4]

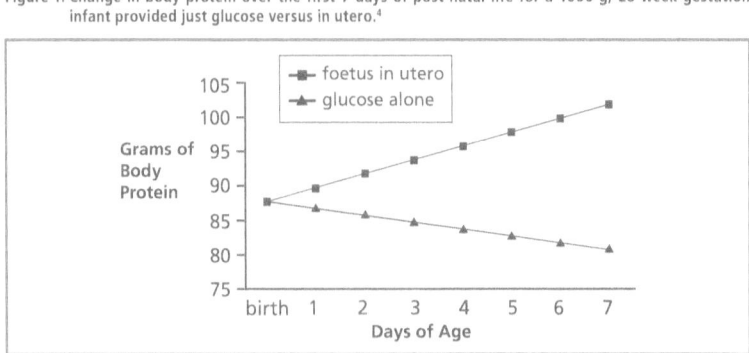

Reprinted from Seminars in Perinatology, Vol 27(4), Dusick AM, et al., Growth failure in the preterm infant: can we catch up?, Pages 302-310, © 2003, with permission from Elsevier.

Initiating TPN early but limit the duration

Importance of early TPN

The European Society for Paediatric Gastroenterology, Hepatology and Nutrition (ESPGHAN) Committee on Nutrition considers the goal for caring for premature infants as obtaining a functional outcome similar to term infants.[6] Part of this goal is to prevent nutritional deficits through early and aggressive parenteral and enteral nutrition.[7]

Poor growth is common in VLBW and extremely low birth weight (ELBW) infants. The US National Institute of Child and Human Development reveals that 16% of ELBW infants are small for gestational age (SGA) at birth, but by 36 weeks, the rate increases to 89%.[4] At 18 to 22 months corrected age, the weights, lengths, and head circumferences of 40% of these infants were still at the 10th percentile.[4] Poor growth may also lead to poor neurodevelopment outcomes. Poor head growth in VLBW infants results in lower mental development index (MDI) at ages 15–20 months[8,9] and lower academic abilities later at school age. Early parenteral nutrition has been shown to improve weight at discharge or at 36 weeks post-menstrual age by almost 15 g.[10] There was a reduction of 3–3.5% in weight loss in infants given early parenteral nutrition.[10] Among VLBW infants who established full enteral feeds by week 2 of life, the infants who received parenteral nutrition had higher weight gain and head growth than those who were not given parenteral nutrition.[11]

Earlier introduction of TPN as well as a more aggressive advancement are effective and safe, even in the smallest and most immature infants.[12] There were no risk of sepsis, NEC, chronic lung disease (CLD), intraventricular haemorrhage (IVH), or cholestasis.[10] There are, however, risks with prolonged TPN.

Limit duration: risks associated with prolonged TPN

TPN complications include infections such as sepsis, bacteraemia, and fungaemia, mechanical issues such as venous thrombosis and superior vena cava syndrome, and metabolic problems such as fluid overload and hypoglycaemia or hyperglycaemia, and other complications such as cholestasis.[13] From the author's clinical experience TPN is consciously targeted to be limited to within a 2-week mark to minimise exposure to the risk of these complications. Adopting the approach of early introduction of MEF and a dependence on breast milk use seemed to facilitate this more successfully. Thus to reduce the burden from these complications, TPN should be kept as short as possible. It is weaned gradually while enteral feeding is advanced. However, TPN should not be ceased abruptly before enteral feeding reaches 120 ml/kg/day, and preferably only when feed volume reaches 150 ml/kg/day in infants without fluid restriction.

Components of parenteral nutrition

TPN is the formulation of nutritional components such as carbohydrates, amino acids, lipids including essential fatty acids, electrolytes, vitamins, minerals, trace elements, water, and other additives that is delivered to a newborn infant intravenously. Previously individualised compounding based on the needs of each individual infant was the mainstay regime. Recently, standardised compounding is gaining acceptance based on favourable compatibilities, cost, and efficiency. Units have to examine which method is best suited to their own needs within their constraints or limitations. Standardised regimen of TPN is based on the principle of "standard" protein, fluids, and electrolytes for different days of postnatal age.[14] In the NICU of Universiti Kebangsaan Malaysia Medical Centre (UKMMC), a "married" standardised-individualised approach is adopted. The example of this regime is referred to in the Appendix.

Keeping the right balance of glucose

In the first few days of life, 4–6 mg/kg/min of glucose should be given and subsequently increased to 8 mg/kg/min.[15;16] However, ELBW infants should be started at 8–10 mg/kg/min.[16] This is called glucose infusion rate (GIR). When glucose is insufficient, a preterm infant with inadequate glycogen storage can easily become hypoglycaemic. On the other hand, over infusion with glucose, can often lead to hyperglycaemia. The very preterm infants may not be able to tolerate excessive sugar, often leading to hyperglycaemia. This is particularly so if the infant is also growth restricted. In fact, the more growth retarded they are, the more insensitive they are to insulin, similar to patients with diabetes. In clinical practice, when the sugar levels are high, physicians should reduce the infant's sugar intake. However, when the sugar is reduced, the infants will then not have sufficient calories for nutrient accretion and growth. Using high protein early on may actually help with an infant's tolerance to sugar. Protein facilitates the taking up of sugar, thus reducing the insensitivity of the cells to insulin and subsequently the problem of hyperglycaemia.[17] Another reason for hyperglycaemia in these infants is an immature pancreas, resulting in insulin not being readily secreted. One solution for this condition is to provide insulin temporarily, which may be the alternative to reducing the amount of sugar that limits the caloric needs of an infant for a positive energy balance.

Prioritising protein

Protein is important for the maintenance of tissue and growth, and crucial for the production of enzymes, hormones, immune factors, and albumin, as well as for cell transport. As protein has short and long-term effects, optimum intake is pivotal, especially for the growth and development of preterm infants. Higher protein intake in ELBW infants was shown to improve their head growth at 18 months corrected age.[18] Higher protein intake in the first few days of life accelerated weight gain in low birth weight (LBW) neonates.[19] Every 1 g/kg/day increase in protein intake during the first week of an ELBW infant's life, was associated with an 8.2 points increase in Bayley MDI at 18 months.[20]

It is difficult to determine the actual normal values for protein profiles and growth in the preterm infants. Standard values are based on intrauterine growth rates and/or growth rates of healthy preterm infants fed adequate amounts of breast milk to mimic intrauterine growth rates (protein intake of 2.7–3.5 g/kg/day with at least 80 non-protein kcal/kg/day to mimic intrauterine accretion).[21] The American Academy of Pediatrics in 1998 estimated that a preterm infant with a birth weight of < 1200 g would require 4 g/kg/day of protein and infants weighing between 1200–1800 g would require about 3.5 g/kg/day.[22] The ESPGHAN recommends 4.0–4.5 g/kg/day of protein intake for infants of birth weight up to 1000 g, and 3.5–4.0 g/kg/day for infants weighing 1000–1800 g.[6]

VLBW infants should be started on amino acid solutions within 1–2 hours of birth. The smallest, sickest preterm infants can tolerate parenteral protein and are more likely to retain positive nitrogen balance if started early.[23] Early initiation of amino acid resulted in better parenteral amino acid intake within the first 5 days of life followed by better growth outcomes (Figure 2).[18] If the preterm infants had remained in the womb, protein accretion for a foetus during the later part of gestation is around 2 g/kg/day.[24] Obligatory protein losses are approximately 0.7 g/kg/day and more if we account for the losses from skin and breathing when extrauterine. With the basal energy expenditure of the relatively stable ELBW infant during the first week of life, 60–80 kcal/kg/day is insufficient to support growth.[25] Protein accretion increases linearly with amino acid intake of 0.5 to 4.0 g/kg/day in the presence of adequate non-protein energy. Approximately 1.5 g/kg/day of amino acid with 30–40 kcal of energy would provide a positive protein balance.[4] Initiating amino acid at 1.5 g/kg/day within 24 hours of birth was well tolerated with no report of adverse effects.[26] Approximately 3.5 g of amino acid parenterally with non-protein energy intake (90 kcal/kg/day) is equivalent to the in utero protein accretion rates that support growth and positive nitrogen balance.[4] As preterm infants experience a higher rate of protein turnover and breakdown because of their immaturity, concomitant illnesses and the very rapid rate of growth and protein accretion, this rate of protein supply is currently the recommended standard of care. Complications such as hyperammonaemia and metabolic acidosis are considered historical concerns which may be related to the previously less refined manufacturing processes and balances in the composition of amino acid, and not the protein amount itself.[27] On this note, some may start with higher protein even from day 1 but the NEON (Nutritional Evaluation and Optimisation in Neonates) trial recently published states that there was no difference in growth with high immediate protein in TPN (3 g/kg/day) compared to the moderate approach commencing at 1.5 g/kg/day. In fact, head circumference was smaller in the higher protein group.[28]

Figure 2. Mean daily quantity of parenteral amino acid over the first 20 days of life in subjects with daily parenteral feeding. This was associated with significantly better growth outcomes at 36 week of post-menstrual age.[18]

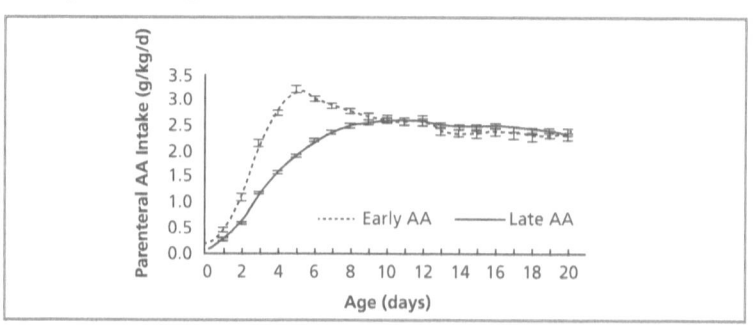

Reprinted from The Journal of Pediatrics, Vol 148(3), Pointdexter BB, et al., Early provision of parenteral amino acids in extremely low birth weight infants: Relation to growth and neurodevelopmental outcome, Pages 300-305, © 2006, with permission from Elsevier.

Lipids are important

Lipids are a source of long-chain polyunsaturated fatty acids (LCPUFAs), which are important for brain and visual development. The ESPGHAN recommends up to a maximum of 3–4 g/kg of parenteral lipid per day, which includes 0.25 g/kg of linoleic acid per day for preterm infants to prevent deficiency in essential fatty acids.[29] As a nutrient with a dense caloric content, lipids are capable of delivering energy in small volumes. This is critical for small infants whose total volume of fluids are restricted, especially when they are sick. As an important nutrient for infants, lipids should be started simultaneously with the other macronutrients (glucose and protein). Traditionally, many practitioners are cautious in using lipids early as they perceived lipid as the primary contributor to or aggravating sepsis. This notion is quite unfounded as essential fatty acids are necessary in the repair of cell injury, particularly in making new cell membranes.

However, lipids may impede coagulation and platelet function, thus it should be used with caution in certain situations. Excessive lipid, may be poorly metabolised especially by sick preterm infants. Nevertheless in sepsis, lipids should only be reduced accordingly instead of ceased entirely. Currently, most centres do not routinely measure triglyceride (TG) levels as done previously. The author's personal practice is to measure TG levels only when preterm infants requiring full TPN are sick or on intensive respiratory support. In these instances, lipids are titrated accordingly, keeping the TG levels below 2.2 mmol/l.

"Traditional" form of intravenous lipids may affect the liver causing cholestasis especially in protracted TPN therapy of more than two weeks. Newer lipids like SMOFlipid® (lipid emulsion containing 15% fish oil together with soy bean, olive and medium chain triglyceride (MCT) oil) may reduce cholestasis,[30] however results from the NEON trial[28] did not show reduction of cholestasis compared to intralipid. The SMOFs besides being reportedly less hepatotoxic, also have MCTs, the form of fatty acids that can be instantly absorbed without being broken down with lipase, an enzyme relatively deficient in the preterm infant. However, as long-chain fatty acids are crucial for brain and visual development, the MCT component should be used judiciously and not be the predominant lipid provided to these infants.

Micronutrients

TPN should also contain electrolytes (potassium, and calcium), vitamins (fat soluble such as vitamins A, D, E and K as well as water soluble ones such as vitamins C, B1, B2, B6, niacin, pantothenic acid and biotin) and microminerals (zinc, copper, chromium, molybdenum, manganese and iodine) to support various metabolic activities.

Infusion routes

The peripheral inserted central catheter (PICC) is the preferred route. However, in many centres without a specified team to perform this procedure, and while waiting for the preterm infant to "stabilise", the infusion route may be relegated through the quicker access of an umbilical venous catheter. However, this method should be only temporary as the risk of infection may be greater and complications from this approach have been reported, e.g. peritoneal extravasation[31] and possibly hepatic necrosis.[32] As an alternative, TPN (if glucose concentration is not more than 12.5%) may sometimes be infused through a peripheral vein temporarily while awaiting proper PICC access.

Inserting the PICC

- Line insertion should be done using sterile techniques.
- The length of insertion is estimated by measuring with a tape from point of entry to site of catheter tip.
- The basilic vein at the antecubital fossa of the upper limb is the preferred site of entry. On the lower limb, the dorsalis or posterior tibialis or saphenous veins are the usual sites.
- The X-ray taken after insertion should preferably be reviewed with a senior medical staff.
- If the catheter tip is not clearly visible, an ultrasound or an X-ray with radio-opaque contrast is used to ensure the tip is outside the heart. Any repositioning of the line should be reconfirmed with a repeat imaging procedure.
- The insertion site is covered with a sterile, preferably visibly clear dressing, and left undisturbed.
- The line insertion, and length as well as the catheter tip siting are documented in the patient's medical record.
- Central line complications are regularly monitored, especially in situations of unexplained hypoglycaemia, thrombophlebitis and catheter-related sepsis. Care should be exercised to avoid advancing the PICC into portal or hepatic veins if accessing from the lower limb veins. The tip should be optimally placed at the superior vena cava (SVC) entry into the right atrium and not in the right atrium if accessed through the upper limbs.
- TPN infusate should be filtered with the appropriate pore-sized filters (for lipids it is 1.2 micrometer and 0.22 micrometer air eliminating for non-lipids) connected in line with the PICC.
- TPN fluid delivery through light opaque tubing connected to the PICC may protect light sensitive nutrients e.g. vitamins (vitamin C) from degradation and limit lipid peroxidation especially as phototherapy is a common practice in the Asian setting.

Readers can gather more information by accessing various readily available online resources, e.g. www.vygon.com.

Figure 3. PICC inserted into the inferior vena cava via the lower limb route.

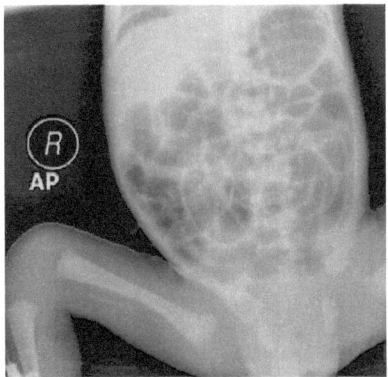

Figure 4. PICC inserted into the superior vena cava via the upper limb approach.

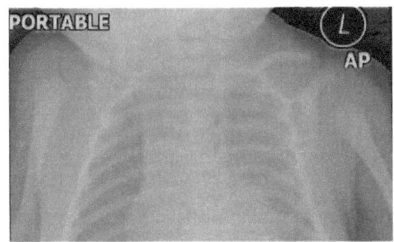

Back to basics: introducing TPN in your centre

The practical tips and information given here are derived from the author's experiences when first introducing TPN support in a new centre and during emergency situations when compounded TPN was not available. While the tips here can be used to guide in initiating TPN support in your own centre, always verify with manufacturers' guide and information, other available hospital protocols and useful online resources such as www.fda.gov (medical devices) for precautions against commonly associated hazards such as the risk of precipitation and instability. Consulting and involving a dedicated pharmacist trained in TPN compounding is highly recommended in a NICU setting.

Preparing parenteral nutrition solutions

Centres with no compounding or a pharmacist to support this, may engage in providing some basic form of TPN by acquiring the raw ingredients and sourcing the macronutrients from major TPN manufacturers such as Fresenius Kabi and Baxter.

Standard parenteral glucose drips, amino acid solutions, and the lipids are drawn individually into three separate syringes in a clean room (preferably under laminar flow or in a Hepa-filter enclosure) and then infused separately via a manifold or three-way stopcock connected to a single PICC line or through alternative intravenous access such as multi-lumen catheters.

Protein solution e.g. Vaminolact® (Kabi); if fluid volume is a limiting factor in the very small infant, use 10% (10 g/100 ml) protein

Otherwise, the usual preparation contains about 6.5 g amino acid/100 ml

Supply at least 1.5 g/kg to avoid catabolism

In a 1 kg infant, it would be 1.5/6.5 x 100 ml

Lipid e.g. SMOFlipid® (Kabi) or Intralipid 20% (choose 20% lipids for optimal phospholipid delivery) i.e. 20 g lipid/100 ml

To supply about 0.5 g lipid as minimum for essential fatty acid = 0.5/20 x 100 ml

Dextrose e.g. Dextrose 10% used to deliver a glucose infusion rate (GIR) of the minimum of 4 mg/kg/min up to the average of 6 mg/kg/min during the first 48 hours of life.

At 5 mg/kg/min,

= 5 x 1 x 60 x 24/1000 ÷ 10 g/100 ml

= (GIR in mg/1000) x (weight in kg) x 60 min x 24 hours ÷ glucose concentration (g%).

= volume of glucose infusate

If compounding is not available or too expensive, centres may opt for a standardised rather than individualising the use of TPN. In an individualised approach, TPN is ordered for each infant based on his needs (volume of fluid needed plus specific nutrient requirements). In the standardised approach, the fluid and nutrient delivery is standardised by days (Day 1, Day 2, etc.). However, sterility in individualised preparation raises concerns about TPN- related sepsis. Also, as minerals such as calcium and phosphorus are necessary in the longer term use, stability of additives in the TPN solution and accuracy during compounding are some contentious issues debated. Various studies are currently emerging in an attempt to resolve these differences.

In the author's practice, a combination of both approaches are used with a six-day standard regimen (see Appendix 1).[33] A pharmacist usually fine-tunes the solutions according to an infant's requirements if necessary. A centre with no TPN- compounding pharmacists or facility should perhaps opt for a standardised regime. Use filters to reduce the risk of infections and inadvertent air or other particulates when infusing the TPN. In the author's practice, the delivery lines are also opaque to reduce light exposure on the TPN to avoid degeneration of light sensitive vitamins and macronutrients such as lipids from peroxidation.

- Fat soluble vitamin (Vitalipid®, Kabi) and water soluble vitamins (Soluvit®, Kabi) (1 ml/kg each) are included together in the lipid drawn syringe. This syringe should be wrapped with opaque foil as some of the vitamins are light sensitive and can be degraded.
- The minerals and electrolytes (Peditrace™, calcium, magnesium and phosphate - 1 ml/kg each) are included together in the glucose- or protein- drawn syringe. Peditrace™ is a solution containing zinc chloride, cupric chloride, manganese chloride, sodium selenite, sodium fluoride and potassium iodide. Organic phosphate should be used to reduce precipitation (especially when higher concentration of calcium is used). For sodium, opt for acetate instead of chloride as small infants are unable to tolerate the chloride load and may result in metabolic acidosis. Also, sodium is usually omitted in the first few days of life because newborn infants have positive sodium balance. Likewise, potassium may be avoided until the infant begins to diurese usually after 48 hours.

Monitoring

Administrating parenteral nutrition can result in metabolic, mechanical (catheter migration and thrombosis) and septic complications. Therefore, assessing these infants prior to starting TPN and close monitoring while receiving TPN are crucial. For metabolic monitoring, laboratory support is necessary in the form of periodic testing of electrolytes, blood urea, creatinine, total calcium, phosphorus, bilirubin, alanine transaminase, alkaline phosphatase, albumin and glucose levels. Most of these tests are done daily, until stable levels have been achieved. Once the TPN delivery rate has stabilised, the testing for these parameters are done less frequently. The infants should also be monitored for their growth by measuring the weight, length and head circumference.

Key points summary

- The majority of preterm infants cannot establish enteral feeds immediately after birth thus they are given nutrients parenterally from Day 1 of life as a crucial nutritional intervention.
- Centres taking care of VLBW infants should have adequate TPN support for early and optimal nutrient delivery to this high risk group of infants.
- Basic TPN support can be made available in most NICU, even in low resource centres as long as some basic monitoring and strict aseptic precautions during preparation is adhered to.
- Parenteral nutrition is the cornerstone of nutrient delivery before enteral feeding could be established in the preterm infant, and is deemed a nutritional emergency intervention.
- TPN should be initiated within the first 24 hours of life in the preterm especially the extremely and very LBW infants.
- The minimum protein of 1.5 g/kg/day is required to avoid catabolism.
- Protein is recommended to start at 3 g/kg/day and advance to 4.5 g/kg/day especially in the ELBW.
- Lipids should not be sidelined and at least 0.5 g/kg/day should be commenced from Day 1 to provide essential fatty acids.

Chapter 2

Early enteral nutrition and feeding strategies for the preterm infant during the acute period of illness

- Fook-Choe Cheah -

What is known on this topic?

- Initiating early enteral feeding in preterm infants is associated with earlier full enteral establishment of feeds, more rapid weight gain, and earlier discharge from hospital.
- In addition, with early enteral nutrition, the infant will require shorter duration of total parenteral nutrition (TPN), thus limiting TPN-related complications.

What this chapter adds?

- Emphasises that enteral feeding for premature infants should be initiated as soon as possible via a proposed minimal enteral feeding (MEF) strategy and advancement, to different groups of at risk infants.
- Breast milk is the choice starter-feed for better tolerance and a lower risk of necrotising enterocolitis (NEC) in all cases.
- Early initiation of enteral feeds is not associated with significantly greater risk of feeding intolerance or NEC.
- Gastric residual volume assessment, often viewed too carefully with no other ominous gastrointestinal (GI) danger signs can be an impediment to successful initiation and early establishment of enteral feeds.

Introduction

Feeding intolerance is common in preterm infants. Almost all of the feeding intolerance among premature infants occur when feeding is initiated within 24 hours of life but tolerance to enteral feeding appears to improve in the following 24 hours. The risk of NEC, following feeding intolerance also raises fear and results in practitioners delaying the feeding of the preterm infant.[34] Feeding of preterm infants is sometimes delayed up to Day 5–7 of life. However, fasting during this early neonatal period may actually be detrimental, increasing the risk of nosocomial infections possibly as a result of gut colonisation by pathogenic bacteria and bacterial translocation. Fasting also has a negative effect on the intestinal immune maturation, motility as well as on the secretory immunoglobulin A (IgA) production.[35]

Early versus delayed enteral feeding

The question that many practitioners ask and the issue frequently raised: if preterm infants especially those who are small for gestational age (SGA) with abnormal umbilical artery flow are at risk for NEC, should early enteral feeding within the first few days after birth be preferably avoided? As even an immature gut can respond to feeding with organised contractions and release of intestinal hormones, early enteral feeding is a logical crucial precedence to reaching full enteral feeding for these infants during the early neonatal period.[36] Early establishment of enteral nutrition will also reduce the dependency on TPN and TPN related complications such as cholestasis and infection. This is especially important for centres that do not have adequate TPN support facilities. Although preterm infants may be at greater risk for feeding intolerance and NEC, a Cochrane review showed no statistically significant increase in NEC in infants who were given early enteral feeds compared to those who were given delayed feeding (more than 5–7 days after birth); and some of the trials in this review did include growth-restricted infants with evidence of abnormal umbilical artery flow.[34] One of these trials was a large study involving 404 preterm infants with intrauterine growth retardation (IUGR) and also abnormal antenatal Doppler studies, from 54 hospitals across the UK and Ireland.[35] This study found growth-restricted preterm infants to be able to achieve full enteral feeding earlier when enteral feeds was introduced early. There also appears to be no increased risk of NEC with early introduction.[37]

In an analysis of the author's own practice, infants who were given enteral feeds within 12 hours of life had lower feeding intolerance (10%) than infants whose enteral feed was initiated after 48 hours of life (25%).[33] This positive effect of an early stimulation of the gut suggests that stable premature SGA infants should be started on enteral feeding as soon as possible.

MEF to prime the immature gut

Instead of delaying feeds in preterm infants, an immediate start with very low volumes of milk should be introduced to encourage gut maturation. This is known as MEF, trophic feeding, gut priming or hypocaloric feeding. With MEF, the feeding tolerance of a preterm infant may be enhanced with the time taken to achieve full enteral feeds reduced.[35] Studies have found that MEF was not associated with higher rates of NEC compared with delayed feeding.[34] Prolonged periods of fasting was associated with a delay in mucosal growth, mucosal atrophy and abnormal secretion of trophic hormones in both humans and animals.[35] Enteral nutrition, even in minimal quantities, encourages the growth of the intestinal mucosa. In addition, MEF increases hormone production, which stimulates intestinal motility.[34] In the author's neonatal unit as well as in Singapore National University Hospital, the feed volumes for preterm infants at risk of NEC are 1 ml 6 hourly (H), 1 ml 3H and 1 ml 2H over the first three days of life. Tolerance is partly guided by gastric residual volumes (GRV). Depending on birth weight, GRV of 2–3 ml while on MEF is considered safe. GRV especially partially digested milk (curd) should not be viewed over-cautiously as a sign to discontinue feeds in the absence of other abdominal signs. Colostrum is the best choice for MEF.

Advancing enteral feeds

Enteral feeds are given at prescribed volumes at scheduled intervals but may vary depending on the neonatal intensive care unit (NICU) practice or the infant risk group.[38] An example of feed advancement is shown in Figure 5. If an infant is able to tolerate the first 1 ml, the intervals may be shortened until the minimum of two hours to gauge if the tolerance continues. It is recommended that the volume in feed advancement not be more than 20 ml/kg/day for the extremely low birth weight (ELBW) infants. Larger volumes may lead to feeding intolerance and NEC especially in the IUGR infant with abnormal Doppler flow (Abnormal Doppler Enteral Prescription Trial -ADEPT).[39] A Cochrane review revealed that there were no effects in the incidence of NEC between infants on slow advancement of feeds (daily increments of 15 to 20 ml/kg) and those who were advanced faster (30 to 35 ml/kg). However, the studies in this review had very few infants who weighed less than 1 kg[40] and as such it is prudent to be more cautious in feed advancement for the smaller infants (< 1 kg at birth) and gestation of < 29 weeks.

The SIFT (Speed of Increasing Milk Feeds trial) which is being completed will throw light on whether to advance feeds by 18 ml/kg/day or 30 ml/kg/day for the VLBW (< 1500 g) infants and those who are preterm, < 32 weeks gestation. The results of this study will hopefully indicate the optimal increment in feeds for this at risk group in terms of growth and safety.[41]

Figure 5. A model flowchart on enteral feeding

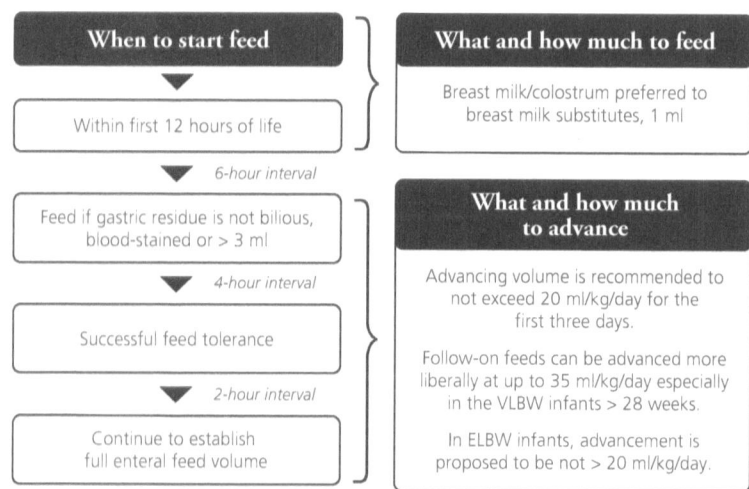

The Singapore National University Hospital is more conservative in their practice when advancing feeds in view of their rates of NEC.[42] In their risk-based feeding protocol, the rate of feed advancement for infants less than 1 kg (extremely low birth weight; ELBW) or ≤ 28 weeks gestation is 10 ml/kg/day till full feeds. For larger very low birth weight (VLBW) infants, the rate is increased to 20 ml/kg/day after Day 7. Other risk factors for NEC will also be factored in when advancing feeds for the individual infant, e.g. with absent or reversed end diastolic blood flow, perinatal hypoxia-ischaemia, significant hypotension and of multiple pregnancies. Frequency of feeding will be converted from 2 hourly to 3 hourly when full feeds (150–180ml/kg/day) are achieved and the infant's weight is more than 1600 g.

Intermittent bolus feeding versus continuous infusion

Due to the distension of the stomach in a small infant from pressurised gases when receiving respiratory support, volume of feeding may be decreased to avoid regurgitation or spills. One way to overcome this is to have smaller volume feeds with shorter intervals, or infusing feeds over half-to-one hourly rather than a fast bolus of less than 20 minutes. Infusion feeding is also associated with less frequent desaturation in the very small infants who are on respiratory support. Some practitioners put these infants on routine continuous infusion feeding but this approach does not have sufficient evidence to warrant as the standard of care.

A Cochrane review has shown a difference between continuous milk feeding and intermittent bolus feeding in terms of time to achieve full feeds and the incidence of NEC.[40] Another review of studies was also in favour of continuous milk feeding, concluding that this may lead to a faster establishment of full enteral feeding in addition to reducing the risk of aggravating hypoxic-ischaemic gut damage in preterm SGA infants.[43] Even with "continuous infusion", the author's practice is to allow about 0.5–1 hour of rest at the end of the infusion in a 2 hourly cycle if possible. This may enhance digestion by enzymes and promote the more physiological response in relation to the surge in gut hormones.[44,45]

Intermittent gavage feeding is preferred over continuous feeds as the former is less dependent on additional medical equipment like perfusion pumps. Intermittent gavage feeding at 2–3 hourly intervals allows for close observation of feeding tolerance, especially during the initial "wait and see" acceptance phase of feed introduction. Continuous feeds however may be useful for infants with significant gastro-oesophageal reflux (GER) or abdominal distension with splinting of the diaphragm in the very small infant on respiratory support such as continuous positive airway pressure (CPAP). When continuous feeds are used, the perfusor pump should be at a lower level from the infant position and the tubing should be as short as possible so as to allow the entire delivery of the less dense milk fat without these getting stuck to the sides of the tubing. The set of tubing should be changed preferably every 4 hours as residual milk in the tubing may become stale at room temperature over this period of time.

Milk of choice

Breast milk is the first choice[46] particularly when it has been shown to be easily digested and more tolerated when introduced early. In the author's practice, breast milk is often unavailable. A breast milk substitute with low osmolarity is used as starter feeds as some studies associated high osmolarity with vomiting/feeding intolerance. The lower osmolarity ready to feed (RTF) milk substitute available in the author's practice setting is a Preterm 22 kcal/oz formula (P22) which is often used in this instance until the infant has achieved 30% of his enteral requirement. Mihatsch et al. has reported better feed tolerance in infants fed with semi-elemental breast milk substitute with low osmolarity.[47] However, for infants with no access to breast milk, the use of donor breast milk should be explored, especially if it has been shown to be associated with less NEC than breast milk substitutes.[46] In the author's practice, we opt for RTF milk substitutes when breast milk is unavailable as RTF in liquid form is sterile in a bottle. It is conceivably cost-beneficial in the long-term with reduced staffing needed for milk preparation and the risk of infections from contamination during preparation using milk powder, which itself is not sterile. Although it is arguable that the GI tract is not sterile, extra precaution may be necessary in feeding the preterm infant as their gut is not mature in defences and may be more susceptible to pathogenic colonisation and possibly nosocomial infections.

Evaluating gastric residuals

Previously, practitioners were quite meticulous in tracking the volumes of gastric residuals, taking these as signs of feeding intolerance and even NEC. In the author's opinion, only two conditions can raise the red flag - bilious (dark green) aspirates that can be an indicator of a GI emergency such as malrotation/volvulus and blood-stained or coffee ground aspirate indicative of a possible bleeding process. Milk curd is normally not a cause of concern and could be fed back to the infant. However, if the residuals are blood-stained or bilious, check for underlying causes. Blood stains could be attributed to swallowed blood-stained amniotic fluid, bleeding diathesis or medications such as ibuprofen, which may induce gastric irritation, or even trauma that are mechanically related such as from feeding tube insertion. In bile-stained residuals, check to see whether the feeding tube is too far down into the duodenum. Persistent bilious residuals could be a sign of malrotation, which is a surgical emergency. Blood-stained amniotic fluid in gastric residuals normally occur during the first 24-48 hours after birth. This is benign. Often, the cause is attributed to delivery in mothers with abruptio placentae. An Apt test (refer to end of this chapter about the Apt test) can be easily done at the bedside to distinguish this from the pathological causes of blood-stained gastric residuals. The Apt test is principled after the difference in oxidation of the foetal versus adult (maternal) haemoglobin.

In general, an aspirate of < 10% of the original volume is not considered as problematic. Less emphasis is now given in monitoring gastric residues. Being overly dependent on monitoring gastric residuals could pose as an impediment to advancing feeds and successfully establishing enteral feeding in the preterm infant. A correct balance is needed in this regard. One should be mindful that continuous infusion feed may not be physiologically normal in triggering the required surge of hormones e.g. insulin and the potential loss of nutrients is more likely while the milk dwells in the tubing before reaching the infant. Another consideration is the necessary change of milk as it should not be left longer than 4 hours at room temperature each time to avoid the risk of bacterial contamination.

Recently, Torazza et al. reported in a very interesting review about how we are evaluating gastric residuals and proposed that perhaps we should be re-looking into the issue of its assessment during enteral feeding of the preterm infant.[48] They pointed out that this evaluation has been routine without sufficient evidence to prove that the practice actually improves care by preventing complications such as feeding intolerance or NEC. In fact, the procedure in assessing gastric residuals may be detrimental by causing damage or irritation of the gastric mucosa during the aspiration process. Their study has shown no significant difference in the feeding outcomes between infants with and without routine gastric residual assessment.[48] This is an important study to stimulate further trials to evaluate the potential risks and benefits of the routine gastric residual assessment. A feeding algorithm including the evaluation of practice of gastric residuals that they have published earlier is quite pragmatic and useful as a protocol in most NICUs (Figure 6).[49]

Figure 6. Feeding algorithm for preterm infants.

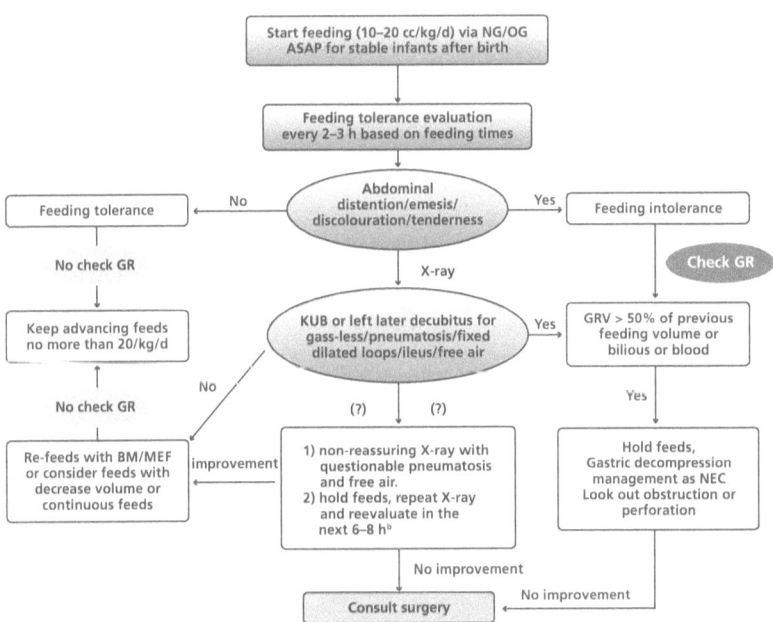

NG = nasogastric; OG = orogastric; ASAP = as soon as possible; h = hourly; GR = gastric residuals; GRV = gastric residual volume; KUB = kidney, ureter and bladder imaging; BM = breast milk; MEF = minimal enteral feeds; NEC = necrotising enterocolitis.
Reprinted from Pediatrics & Neonatology, Vol 55(5), Li Y-F, et al., Gastric Residual Evaluation in Preterm Neonates: A Useful Monitoring Technique or a Hindrance?, Pages 335-340, © 2014, with permission from Elsevier.

Managing feeding intolerance

Feeding intolerance, while it should be recognised early, may also be often "over-diagnosed" and easily used as an excuse to stop or advance feeds. When there is such a problem, attempt to modify the enteral feeding first instead of stopping it abruptly. Green gastric residues in VLBW infants may indicate physiological duodeno-gastric reflux. If there are no other associated gastrointestinal tract (GIT) signs such as abdominal distension or significant illness, feeding should not be stopped.[50] On the other hand, feeding intolerance can be an early sign of NEC; but only if this diagnosis is highly likely should feeding be stopped immediately. In such circumstances, look for other features of NEC in abdominal X-rays, stool for occult blood, and blood test for inflammatory markers, e.g. C-reactive protein (CRP).

Managing infants on nasal CPAP support may sometimes complicate enteral feeding because of gaseous gastric distension ("CPAP belly"). This entity is observed as a distended abdomen with occasional peristaltic loops of bowel visible, no red or "shiny" skin of the abdominal wall, with normal bowel sounds. Intermittent decompression between feeds through the feeding tube can alleviate this problem.

Feeding intolerance may also be related to intestinal dysmotility and lack of bowel movement, which can delay the establishment of enteral feeding.[34] Some infants may benefit from periodic use of glycerin suppositories or enema. Early enteral nutrition was associated with acceleration of meconium passage that may actually improve early feeding tolerance in ELBW infants.[51]

The majority of premature infants do not have a fully developed anti-reflux mechanism. Reflux of stomach contents into the oesophagus, is often in a mild form, and a physiologically normal process in the preterm infant. Rarely, the acidity and quantity of the gastric residuals can make it clinically relevant,[52,53] with complications such as frequent desaturation and even aspiration pneumonia. Smaller volumes and longer infusion time may be corrective in such situations. Anti-reflux therapy should only be used judiciously. Acid reducing agents may be associated with greater bacterial colonisation of the gut and potentially causing sepsis. Feed thickeners are best avoided as they have been reported to be associated with NEC.[54]

Key points summary

- Delaying enteral feeds has negative effects on the preterm infant such as a longer stay in the NICU, slower weight gain, and increased risk of late onset sepsis (LOS).[40,55]
- Early enteral feeding within the first 12–24 hours, especially with breast milk is not associated with increased feeding intolerance or NEC.
- MEF (5–15 ml/kg/day) is an important strategy to prime the immature gut for improved feed tolerance and towards establishing full enteral nutrition and achieving a more rapid weight increase.
- Colostrum/breast milk is the first choice of feeds when initiating feeding enterally. Advancing feeds can be up to 35 ml/kg/day in stable infants but increase cautiously to not more than 20 ml/kg/day for the more at risk group of infants such as the extremely preterm (less than 28 weeks gestation) or ELBW (less than 1000 g birth weight) and preterm SGA infants with compromised gut circulation.
- Consider donor breast milk if mother's own milk is not available. The last alternative option is breast milk substitutes. Lower osmolarity breast milk substitutes may be better tolerated for some infants.
- Many episodes of increased/abnormal gastric residuals may be transient and not pernicious in nature. Identify the underlying cause and modify enteral feeds rather than ceasing it abruptly.

Apt test[56]

The Apt test or Alkali Denaturation Test by Apt and Downey is a simple and quick screening procedure for detecting blood in gastric aspirate or vomitus. It is able to differentiate between blood originating from the neonatal GIT and swallowed maternal blood. This is based on the fact that foetal haemoglobin (Hb F) has a greater resistance to alkaline denaturation compared to adult haemoglobin (Hb A).

Procedure:

- Fresh gastric aspirate or vomitus is obtained.
- Each sample is mixed with an equal volume of distilled water.
- This mixture is centrifuged for 10 minutes at 1000 x g in a bench centrifuge.
- The resulting supernatant will be pink in colour.
- The available supernatant is then mixed with 1 mL of 1% sodium hydroxide (NaOH) for each 5 mL of supernatant.
- If the supernatant remains pink for more than 2 minutes, there is presence of Hb F.
- If it turns yellow/brown within 2 minutes, there is a predominance of Hb A.

Chapter 3

Strategies towards successful breastfeeding and individualising nutritional needs of the preterm infant

- Fook-Choe Cheah -

What is known on this topic?

- Breast milk is recommended for preterm infants due to its various benefits, especially immunoprotective properties.
- Breast milk is generally deficient in calories for the rapidly growing preterm infants, as such fortification of breast milk is a necessity to supplement this extracaloric requirement.

What this chapter adds?

- Practical strategies to promote the use of breast milk, and lactational support to mothers of preterm infants during their stay in the neonatal intensive care unit (NICU) in a diverse socio-economic and cultural environment.
- Discusses the variability of breast milk content that could affect growth, and strategies to overcome deficiency of nutrients such as in fore versus hind milk.
- Bedside analysis of breast milk to facilitate individualisation of nutritional support for optimal growth of the preterm infant.
- Discusses evidence in the practice of human milk fortification, increasing growth rates and enhancing neurodevelopmental outcomes.

Introduction

Breast milk is the milk of choice to feed the preterm infant because of its vital roles in immune development and gastrointestinal (GI) maturation. The advantages of breast milk are irrefutable; in fact, exclusive breastfeeding is recommended for term infants up to 6 months, to be supplemented with other foods from this age on, and breastfeeding preferably is continued until at least 2 years of age. This also applies to preterm infants although specific nutrient enrichment/fortification is needed. In addition, challenges inherently encountered in diminished rates of preterm infants who are breastfed,[57] are necessarily addressed to maximise the benefits of breastfeeding.

The physiology of lactation

Lactogenesis, commencing in mid-pregnancy, begins to transform the mammary gland towards achieving peak lactation sometime after full-term. By the second or third trimester, the mammary gland is equipped to secrete milk but high circulating levels of progesterone and oestrogen inhibit the secretion of milk. This stage before delivery is known as lactogenesis I.

Around the time of delivery, blood flow, oxygen, and glucose uptake increase. The concentration of citrate also increases sharply. When the placenta is removed, the source of progesterone during pregnancy is removed; thus milk secretion is initiated. At this stage of lactogenesis (also known as lactogenesis II), the mammary gland receives hormonal signals, in response to stimulation of the nipple and areola. These hormonal signals are relayed to the central nervous system; creating a cyclical process of milk synthesis and secretion. This process, which is termed as lactation, occurs with the aid of prolactin and oxytoxin. These two hormones act independently on different cellular receptors but their actions in combination are important for lactation. Prolactin is produced by lactotrophic cells in the anterior pituitary and this hormone activates mammary gland epithelial cell PRL (prolactin) receptors. Prolactin also stimulates mammary glandular ductal growth and epithelial cell proliferation, thus inducing milk protein synthesis. Oxytoxin, the other important hormone, is released when the infant begins suckling on the breast. This suckling stimulates touch receptors around the nipple and areola; and the impulses that are created activate the dorsal root ganglia via the intercostal nerves. Oxytoxin causes the contraction of myoepithelial cells that line the ducts of the breast. When stimulated, these smooth muscle-like cells expel milk from the alveoli into ducts and subareolar sinuses, which will then empty through a nipple pore.

There are several factors that inhibit lactogenesis II in mothers of preterm infants that contribute to the impediment of full lactational potential (Figure 7). Antenatal steroids such as betamethasone which is given to pregnant women expecting preterm delivery, can prematurely inhibit lactation. In addition, inadequate stimulation in mothers because their preterm infants are sick or physically not adept to suck at the breast, inhibits milk ejection. Furthermore, when mothers are faced with various stresses related to preterm delivery, milk ejection during expressing becomes more difficult. Stress hormones are found to suppress lactation as the increased levels of dopamine and/or norepinephrine will inhibit prolactin synthesis, which will then result in the down-regulation of milk synthesis. In vivo and in vitro studies have also found cortisol to reduce the tight junction permeability in the lactating mammary.[58,59]

Figure 7. The lactation process and how it is inhibited in preterm births

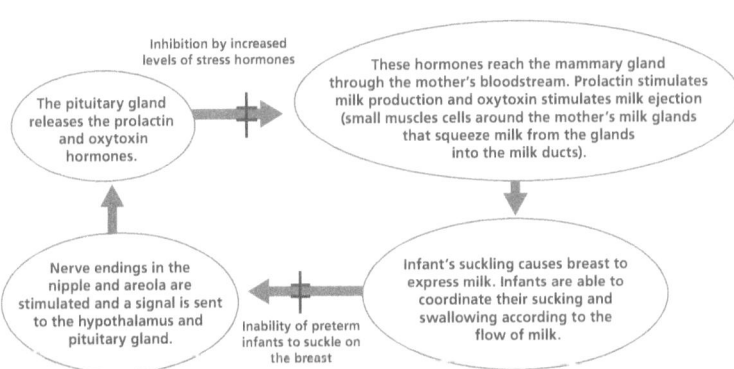

The benefits of using breast milk to feed preterm infants

The biologically active molecules in breast milk promote active and passive stimulation of the immune system,[60] and the right amount of breast milk will ensure the development of an optimal mucosal barrier function in the gut of a newborn.[61,62] Numerous studies have shown breast milk (including donor milk) to reduce necrotising enterocolitis (NEC) compared to breast milk substitutes.[63-65]

In the long-term, breast milk provides immunologic protection against minor infant ills (including otitis media and respiratory tract infections), leading to fewer visits to the paediatrician, hospitalisations, and prescriptions per infant during the first year of life.[66,67]

Babies who were fed with breast milk had more mature visual skills and higher intelligence quotient (IQ) than babies fed with breast milk substitute. This could be attributed to the relatively high levels of long chain polyunsaturated fatty acids (LCPUFAs) in breast milk.

Preterm infants who received breast milk were likely to have better psychomotor, neurological, and cognitive outcomes than infants on breast milk substitute.[68,69]

The World Health Organisation (WHO) recommendation for feeding low birth weight infants is illustrated in figure 8.[70]

Figure 8. The World Health Organization's recommendation for feeding of low birth weight infants.[70]

Best	1. Mother's own breast milk (fresh)	Helps bonding Helps establish lactation
↓	2. Donated fresh preterm milk	Good balance of nutrients (may need supplemental calcium and vitamin D) Prevents infection Easily digested
	3. Donated fresh term mature milk	Prevents infection Easily digested, but lack adequate protein Usually foremilk, so may lack fat
	4. Pasteurised donated breast milk	Easily digested HIV destroyed, anti- infective factors partially lost
	5. Preterm formula	Correct nutrients, but not necessarily easily digestible No anti-infective properties More severe infections
Worst	6. Ordinary formula	Wrong balance of nutrients No anti-infective properties Less optimal growth and development More severe infections Difficult to digest and utilise

Reprinted from International Breastfeeding Journal, 1(26), Arnold LDW, Global health policies that support the use of banked donor human milk: a human rights issue, 2006, with permission from BioMed Central.

Practical issues and considerations in breastfeeding of preterm infants

Logistics and support for mothers

Hospitals that do not have the equipment, staff and logistics for women to breastfeed or express breast milk constitutes a main hurdle in successful breastfeeding of the preterm infant. As the preterm infant will have to remain in the NICU for a significantly long duration in many occasions, the lack of rooming-in facilities in a hospital where the mother and child can be together 24 hours a day will be challenging to transition to full breastfeeding before discharge. The lactation nurse needs to be familiar with the preterm infant's needs to be able to fine-tune or tweak standard processes accordingly.

In addition, social and cultural practices of some communities may limit the mother's access to her preterm infant. The post-partum confinement process, in which the mother stays at home to recuperate, inevitably separates the preterm infant from the mother. In some advanced countries (e.g. in Scandinavian countries), family-centred care has emerged to the forefront by engaging hospitals to be involved in providing the necessary facilities for 24 hours co-bedding with monitoring. Even if there are no limiting cultural practices, in many countries in this region, where large family units exist, many mothers have difficulty going away to the hospital as they have other children to take care of at home. Reaching out to these mothers is, however, crucial; this can be done if community nurses are trained in providing breastfeeding support and the family-centred care concept can be introduced into creche/nurseries built in hospitals to provide the necessary support for the parents and their family.

Financial or transport assistance to enable daily travel between hospital and home to nurse the infant in the absence of family-centred care may be an appropriate interim measure as many mothers depend on the husband's availability to time transportation to the hospital. In addition, public transport may be lacking in many suburban (rural) environment in this region.

Expressed breast milk to feed the preterm infant with immature suckling, swallowing and breathing coordination.

The integration of sucking, swallowing, and breathing is considered an organised behaviour of the young infant; and is critical in achieving safe and successful oral feeding in preterm infants before being allowed discharge to home.

In preterm infants, this coordination is uncoordinated or immature, and infants may have a compromised respiratory system (nasal flaring and tachypnoea between sucking bursts, apnoea, or hypoxaemia). A preterm infant's ability to recover from an oxygen desaturation episode during feeding is dependent on the duration of the breathing period and the ability of the infant to increase ventilation during sucking pause. Oxygen desaturation is common in preterm infants with underlying respiratory problems such as bronchopulmonary dysplasia. Preterm infants have three times more desaturation when bottle fed than with bolus gavage feeding ($p < 0.001$).[71] They may develop significant desaturation which can be effectively reduced by gavage feeding.[71] In the author's practice, infants with such issues will be supplemented with oxygen during feeding times.

Other issues affecting the sucking include the mother's nipple being too big for the infant's mouth, poor latching and technique resulting in cracked nipples, thus impeding success in breastfeeding. If a mother's nipple is too big for the infant's mouth, a nipple shield can be used to reduce the size. The shield can also be useful for mothers with cracked nipples. A speech pathologist can be engaged to help with the sucking and breathing coordination. Non-nutritive sucking or comfort nursing is a way to satiate the infant's need for soothing and bonding during kangaroo mother care (KMC) while the mother and baby learn to establish breastfeeding together. During gavage feeding periods, infants may be allowed to suck on a pacifier or even the nipple during KMC to stimulate the sucking response when milk feeds flow into the stomach.

A preterm infant's inability to suck, coordinate breathing and swallowing mean that mothers would have to express their breast milk for feeding. The only option to feed the infant is through an oro- or nasogastric tube. There are recognisable disadvantages with this method including the reduced absorption of nutrients caused by mechanical issues such as the tube bypassing certain portions of the GI tract, fat particles getting stuck to the walls of the tubing and therefore reducing macronutrients especially fat in breast milk, loss of vitamins through oxidation by air and ambient light, and the occasional spills from gastric distension due to pressurised gas/air from respiratory support such as continuous positive airway pressure (CPAP) or high flow nasal cannula therapy. These are some factors that could contribute to challenges with optimising nutrient delivery and growth of the preterm infant when establishing enteral feeding.

There are some other hazards associated with the use of expressed milk. Bacterial contamination due to unhygienic handling and improper storage have been reported. Theoretically it is not implausible that feeding the immature gut high pathogenic bacterial loads may predispose the infant to infection or even NEC. This is more so when the premature gut has lower colonisation with "good" bacteria (probiotics) secondary to lower gestation and exposure to antibiotics.

Cytomegalovirus transmission concerns from mother to infant through expressed breast milk.

In optimising the use of expressed breast milk (EBM), pasteurisation of breast milk may be an option in countries without donor milk banks implementing inter-patient sharing of milk within the unit, made feasible if there is a standard operating procedure for such transfers to take place.

Breast milk is a potential source of human cytomegalovirus (CMV) infection in preterm infants. The breast milk of mothers who are IgG-positive for CMV may contain the virus by the fourth week after delivery.[72] CMV infection in very immature infants with multiple pre-existing problems, can trigger a severe deterioration of the clinical course and the prolonged need for respiratory support.[73] In order to reduce the infection, breast milk should be frozen at −20°C.[74] In the same paper, it was stated that after 1 night storage, infectivity was reduced by 90%, after 72 hours storage, infectivity reduced by 99% and after 7 days, no infectious virus was detected.[74] The quality of breast milk did not appear to deteriorate significantly after freezing for several days.[75]

There has been reported concerns of breast milk contamination by pathogenic bacteria that may be linked to outbreaks of NEC in preterm infants.[76,77] Although raw breast milk containing various protective antibodies and probiotics are protective against NEC, heavier presence of bacteria, especially gram negative pathogens from contamination has never been really studied as a possible risk factor for NEC. In the study by Cheah et al., EBM from mothers in a NICU in Malaysia contained, in the majority of samples, gram negative bacteria.[78] This may be quite different from skin flora bacteria such as coagulase negative staphylococcus or *Staphylococcus aureus*, reported in centres from temperate countries. Perhaps the hot/humid tropical weather and level of hygiene may contribute to this variation but cultural practices such as limited bathing during confinement may also be an underlying possibility.[77] As such, EBM brought from home may first be cultured routinely to determine if heavy contamination occurs followed by pasteurisation if necessary. If EBM is to be pasteurised, it is imperative to determine if *Bacillus* species is present as this group of bacteria make spores that cannot be killed by pasteurisation. Such milk should be discarded. Centres that believe in routinely pasteurising the EBM before use should ensure proper servicing and maintenance of their in-house pasteurisation apparatus. The quality of breast milk may also be affected with the loss of protective immune factors[79] as well as some nutrients. As for the use of donor human milk in the NICU to take place, regulatory bodies including religious bodies may need to be involved and various social rather than "legal" implications in having an in-house mini milk bank should be considered.

Breastfeeding support for mothers and their infants

The NICU could be a strange, unfamiliar, and intimidating place for mothers. Added with concern for her sick preterm infant, lactation could be negatively affected. Support with encouragement and providing a "homey"/non-threatening environment are important in making breastfeeding a success. A preterm infant may have less respiratory reserve and often has problems with sucking and swallowing, making breastfeeding more challenging as well. Here, nurses and lactational support providers play an important role in educating and emphasising to mothers the merits of breastfeeding while supporting and encouraging them through these difficulties.[80,81] Mothers should be reminded regularly with positive re-enforcement of their important participation and involvement. Fear of handling their infants because of attached/surrounding monitoring tools should be countered by explaining the function of these items and the ways in handling each of them. Mothers should also be empowered to partake actively in KMC, and encouraged to participate in group support together with other breastfeeding mothers.

The 10 steps in promoting breastfeeding of the preterm infant[82,83]

1. Ensure parents have the necessary information to make an informed decision to breastfeed.
2. Guide the mother to establish and maintain milk supply with a target to achieve required volumes/day.
3. Ensure that breast milk management (storage and handling) is done correctly.
4. Establish breast milk feeding procedures and approaches.
5. Encourage skin-to-skin care (KMC).
6. Provide opportunities for non-nutritive sucking at the breast.
7. Manage the transition to the breast.
8. Measure the transfer of milk by determining infant's weight gain.[80]
9. Prepare the infant and the family for hospital discharge.
10. Provide appropriate follow-up care.

Stimulating and maintaining lactation

Breast pumps are primarily used to express milk from the breasts of a lactating woman to be stored and fed later to an infant. Manual expression by hand is also effective with the right technique emphasised (Figure 9). Recently, a randomised trial showed higher fat content in breast milk expressed manually. This energy/caloric advantage may be attributed to more hind milk present when massaging the breast during manual expression.[84] The manual breast pumps are less expensive than electronic breast pumps, but the latter may be preferred by women to pump regularly with their hands free to do other activities. Some breast pumps can aid lactating women with a low milk supply. Medela, a company that produces products and programmes for breastfeeding, introduced a breast pump that simulates the different sucking and pausing rhythms of a newborn infant. Their Symphony® breast pump can be programmed to provide pumping patterns with frequencies of 45 to 125 cycles/min and vacuums of -45 to -273 mm Hg; the applied vacuum was found to have an effect on the amount of milk that was removed of up to 50 to 70 seconds after milk ejection.[85] This apparatus is claimed to be able to stimulate the production of breast milk equivalent to that from mothers of term infants after 6 days.[86]

Figure 9. Manual expression of milk from the breast.

Step 1: Gently massage breast.

 **Step 2**: Put the thumb on top of the area where the areola meets the breast tissue, and place the index finger on the bottom.

Step 3: Push fingers into the chest wall and compress rhythmically until the milk stops spraying.

Step 4: Reposition fingers and thumb (moving like the hands of a clock), and repeat Step 3 several times until all areas are covered.

Step 5: Repeat Steps 1–4 on the other breast.

Studies on the efficacy of different galactogogues, which are used to induce higher lactation and milk production are still inconclusive.[87] One of the more commonly studied and widely used galactogogues is domperidone. In two studies, mothers of preterm infants on domperidone had a steady increase in milk volume and this could be attributed to the stimulation of prolactin secretion.[88] More studies on the efficacy of this drug are needed. There were also some evidence on the use of metoclopramide, fenugreek, asparagus, and milk thistle[87] but efficacy and safety data for these were insufficient.

Donor breast milk

> *Where it is not possible for the biological mother to breastfeed, the first alternative, if available, should be the use of human breast milk from other sources.*
>
> *Human milk banks should be made available in appropriate situations.*
>
> Joint statement by the WHO/United Nations Children's Fund, 1980

When there is inadequate mother's own milk, donor milk through human milk bank, one-to-one sharing, and commercial breast milk chain supply can serve as alternatives. Except for the loss of some antibodies, immune factors and enzymes, pasteurised donor breast milk is similar to a mother's own milk. Nevertheless, the milk needs to be stored and transported properly (see http://www.cdc.gov/breastfeeding/recommendations/handling_breastmilk.htm for how to store and transport donor breast milk).

In human milk banks, expressed breast milk are pooled after collection from pre-screened mothers who have abundant milk supply. The milk is then pasteurised before being used to feed infants who need them. These infants include premature infants whose mothers have insufficient breast milk. Many countries have instituted milk banks, and these include France, United Kingdom, USA, India, China, and the Philippines.

For countries with no milk banks, one-to-one sharing of breast milk is an option, and this is more practical for mothers whose religion forbids the use of milk from an unknown or multiple sources. One-to-one sharing approach, however, has its risks and challenges in terms of the infectious disease status of the donor, storage and pasteurisation. Several Middle Eastern countries have reported this sharing arrangement. The Duchess of Kent Hospital, Tawau, Sabah has also developed a protocol for one-to-one sharing in their NICU.[89] Hospitals need the resources to set up these facilities, if the mothers are unable to do so themselves.

Another option is the use of commercial breast milk suppliers that offer milk-based nutritional products (e.g. Prolacta Bioscience, Inc.), which cater for premature infants in the NICU. The question of ethics, however, arise on whether commercial breast milk supply is similar to the selling of any other biological product such as blood. Quality control and the regulatory process for such establishments need to be monitored and be transparent to the end user.

The need to fortify breast milk for preterm infants

The WHO recommends breast milk over breast milk substitute feeding to the preterm infant but also specifies the need for supplementation.[47] The breast milk caloric energy content is about 20 kcal/oz but the preterm infant will need at least 24 kcal/oz energy content for rapid growth to simulate intrauterine accretion rate. Although breast milk is still preferred as the feed of choice because of the presence of immune and growth factors, the energy content needs boosting.

Another main component of breast milk that is important to highlight is the human milk oligosaccharide (HMO), which has major roles in the prebiotic, immunomodulatory and antimicrobial effects as well as other important biological functions.[90] HMO may offer protection against NEC, and also contributes to visual and brain development.[91] Although the amount and composition of oligosaccharides (OS) vary among women and at different stages of lactation,[92] OS found in cow's milk cannot be matched to the amount and complexity of HMOs.[93] More discussion on HMOs are referred to in Chapter 7 on pro- and prebiotics.

The protein content of breast milk is variable and can be as low as 1.2–1.5 g/100 ml. Preterm infants require at least 2.5–3 times more for tissue "expansion" for anabolism. Protein supplementation of breast milk promotes growth in preterm infants. The effects include increases in weight gain (with a weighted mean difference, WMD of 3.6 g/kg/day, 95% Confidence Interval; CI:2.4 to 4.8 g/kg/day), linear growth (WMD 0.28 cm/week, 95% CI:0.18 to 0.38 cm/week) and head growth (WMD 0.15 cm/week, 95% CI:0.06 to 0.23 cm/week).[94] These outcomes however were primarily short term while long term neurodevelopmental and growth effects have not been sufficiently evaluated.

Infants need vitamin D for bone metabolism, immunity, and prevention against allergies. But as the content of vitamin D is insufficient in breast milk, the American Academy of Pediatrics recommends that every child who is breastfed be given vitamin D supplementation to meet an intake of 400 IU/day.[95] Even in tropical countries such as Malaysia, vitamin D supplementation may be necessary as people tend to stay away from the overbearing sun. Muslim women who wear headgears and long sleeved attire, limit their skin exposure to the sun[96] while darker skin individuals (greater skin melanin interferes with vitamin D synthesis) reportedly have low levels of vitamin D.[97] There are still no guidelines available as to the recommended supplementation of vitamin D in preterm infants. More over, vitamin D levels may vary according to gestation. As the foetus receives majority of its body calcium and phosphorus after week 24 of gestation, preterm infants would require supplementation to improve their bone mineral accretion rates,[98] reducing their risk of metabolic bone disease and improving skeletal growth.

It has also been shown that supplementing breast milk with docosahexaenoic acid (DHA) is beneficial for preterm infants. The European Society of Paediatric Gastroenterology, Hepatology and Nutrition (ESPGHAN) recommends DHA intakes of 12–30 mg/kg/day or 11–27 mg/100 kcal.[22] In one study, a DHA dose of 1% of total fatty acids from Day 2–4 of life increased the Bayley mental developmental index (MDI) scores of preterm infant girls at 18 months of age.[99] In another study with preterm infant boys who were given DHA supplement had less incidence of bronchopulmonary dysplasia.[100]

Fortifying breast milk with human milk fortifiers (HMF) (see Appendix 2) will increase protein, vitamins and minerals to ensure more optimal growth, particularly linear growth in the preterm infant. There are no additional OS, vitamin D or DHA in these current samples of HMFs.

Individualising enteral nutrition to the preterm infant for optimal growth

The composition of breast milk varies among lactating women and even in the same women during different periods of lactation. The composition in the foremilk and hindmilk are also different. For example, though the protein content of breast milk as a whole decreases from early lactation to late lactation period, the hind milk has a higher concentration of fat than fore milk but lower lactose content.[101] Although knowing the specific energy and protein content of breast milk may not make a difference for term infants, it may be important to meet the special needs of the individual preterm infant.[102] There are devices available to measure the levels of creamatocrit (lipid concentration of breast milk), both for home use and in the hospital (Figure 10a). In a study done in the author's practice, milk samples of lactating mothers who delivered prematurely (26–34 weeks gestation) were measured using the creamatocrit machine.[103] The creamatocrit content was positively linked to increasing gestational age but was significantly reduced with pasteurisation.[103]

Recently an automated and more precise instrument that analyses the caloric content of breast milk at the bedside has been introduced, e.g. the MIRIS milk analyser (Figure 10b). Using this method, additional protein could be adjusted to optimise the growth rate. In addition to additional protein in HMF, whey protein concentrate is also added to titrate to the maximum protein recommended. Growth of the preterm infants especially the head circumference of extremely low birth weight (ELBW) infants is more rapid among those babies receiving fortified breast milk that were adjusted with additional whey protein.[104] Other practitioners without access to such milk analyser use a targeted approach based on periodic tests of blood urea (not to exceed 5 mmol/l) as the amount of protein is increased to the maximum recommended. Arslanoglu *et al.* in their study also found a beneficial growth effect with this approach.[105]

Figure 10. Devices to measure the creamatocrit and caloric content of breast milk.

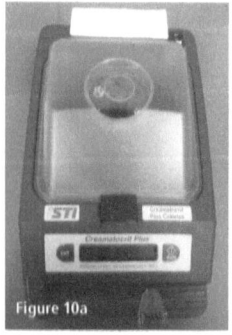
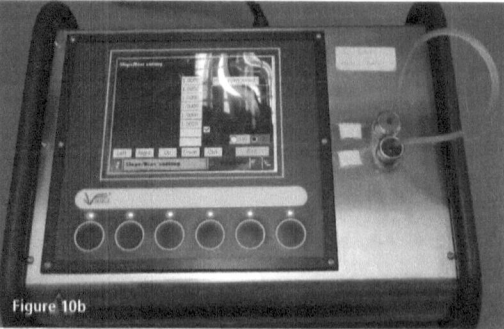

Figure 10a. Figure 10b.

> **Useful resources**
>
> *Centers for Disease Control and Prevention:* Describes the proper handling and storing of breast milk. http://www.cdc.gov/breastfeeding/recommendations/handling_breastmilk.htm
>
> *Medela:* Develops various breastfeeding products for breast care, pumping, collecting milk, breast milk management, and feeding. www.medela.com
>
> *Newborn Individualized Developmental Care and Assessment Program (NIDCAP):* Offers training and certification on supportive care and assessment for preterm newborns and their families in the hospital, and the transition home. http://nidcap.org/en/about-us/our-stories/nidcap.org/en/about-us/our-stories/
>
> *Prolacta Bioscience:* Provides human-milk based nutrition for preterm infants. http://www.prolacta.com/

Key points summary

- Feeding the preterm infant with breast milk is a potent step in significantly reducing NEC.
- Breast milk is preferred to breast milk substitute for its various benefits especially in promoting a healthy immune function and improved neurodevelopmental outcomes, but fortification/supplementation of breast milk with protein and minerals (calcium/phosphorus) are key aspects in optimising growth of the breastfed preterm infant.
- Individualisation with adjusted maximal protein (4.5 g/kg/day) in fortified breast milk may achieve better growth rates especially in head circumference in the very preterm and ELBW infants.
- Mothers of preterm infants require extra lactational support to make breastfeeding successful. Often interim measures and alternatives may be necessary such as in the sharing or the use of donor human milk as well as the use of galactogogues.
- Pathogen transmission in breast milk from mother to the preterm infant requires awareness and surveillance according to the local context with appropriate measures such as freezing and pasteurisation incorporated in protocols as necessary.

Chapter 4

Monitoring and optimising growth of stable preterm infants in the convalescent phase

- Ye-Le Lee & Jiun Lee -

What is known on this topic?

- Early optimal nutritional support and growth is crucial for neurodevelopment, and the time in the neonatal intensive care unit (NICU) is a critical period for preterm infants to catch up on their growth.
- Majority of preterm infants do not achieve catch up growth, and become growth retarded on discharge even at term corrected age.

What this chapter adds?

- Monitoring of growth and recognising growth failure with discussions on strategies and intervention to address growth retardation in the stable preterm infant during convalescence in the NICU.
- Consideration of non-nutritive factors that may result in an infant's growth failure such as improper feeding technique and thermal neutral balance.
- Individualising nutrition with periodic nutrient density monitoring to improve growth outcomes before discharge from hospital.

Introduction

Stable growing preterm infants recovering from their illness while in the NICU offers the best window of opportunity for nutritional intervention to attempt catch-up growth. Although many of them are already on full enteral feeds, a large number of these infants have fallen off the growth centile. If this failure is not overcome, these infants may not be able to reach their growth and cognitive potential. The only way to know if growth is faltering, is to carefully, consistently and regularly monitor their growth parameters (head circumference, length and weight) and conduct some nutritional biochemical analysis. This is also the critical period when parents are encouraged to engage in caring for their child as they learn the skills to take over the care of the infants upon discharge. The catch-up period preferably continues upon discharge with close monitoring and appropriate intervention, as optimising growth within the first two years is paramount in ensuring good neurodevelopmental outcomes.

Post-natal growth failure in premature infants

Very low birth weight (VLBW) infants are faced with a challenging transition to extrauterine life. Respiratory conditions, infections and immature gastrointestinal (GI) function often limit nutritional intake, particularly during the critical first 2-week window of opportunity in nutritional programming. There is also the ever present danger of necrotising enterocolitis (NEC), more so in the extremely and very preterm infants. To achieve growth for VLBW infants approximating foetal weight gain (15 g/kg/day), energy requirements will need to be at least 90–110 kcal/kg/day through the parenteral route or 100–130 kcal/kg/day enterally.[106] This is a rather difficult target, particularly during the early weeks of life, thereby resulting in post-natal growth failure. Singapore National University Hospital's unpublished data confirmed this very common phenomenon (Table 1). At birth, 16.3% were small for gestational age (SGA) (weight < 10th percentile). At 36 weeks post-menstrual age (PMA), more than 81.4% were < 10th percentile, although this improved significantly at 45 weeks (46.5%). These findings were similar to other reports.[107-110]

Table 1: Post-natal growth failure in VLBW infants - National University Hospital cohort 2011

Parameter	At birth	* PMA 36 weeks	* PMA 45 weeks
Weight (g)	1117 (547–1499)	1775 (1050–2381)	3757 (2270–5620)
Length (cm)	36.5 (26.5–42.0)	41.4 (36.0–46.0)	51.0 (42.4–57.0)
Occipital frontal circumference (OFC) (cm)	26.1 (21.0–29.5)	30.3 (27.3–33.5)	36.7 (33.1–39.5)
**SGA (%)	16.3	81.4	46.5

Results in (mean) (range) unless otherwise specified
*PMA = post-menstrual age, **SGA defined as weight < 10th percentile

Early nutritional support and growth during NICU stay have been consistently shown to positively influence neurocognitive outcome.[111-113] Higher energy intake during the first week of life in ill premature infants reduced the risk of morbidities like chronic lung disease (CLD) and late onset sepsis (LOS).[114] Improving post-natal growth is thus crucial and potentially modifiable for ensuring good developmental outcomes.

Special needs group: the preterm SGA infants

The prevalence of growth retardation varies from 20–36%, which may represent selected high-risk pregnancies managed at tertiary centres.[115-117] An SGA state is associated with higher mortality and poorer neurodevelopmental outcomes. The focus in the preterm SGA infant has been not just in achieving normal but more so in catch-up growth.[112] The optimal degree of catch-up growth however has been controversial. There is very good recent data to suggest that excessive catch-up growth puts an infant especially of term gestation, at risk of metabolic syndrome decades later (Barker's hypothesis).[118-120]

The SGA infants in the National University Hospital are fed using the same protocol as non-SGA infants, with similar growth targets, the only difference being a slower advancement of feeds with the hope of minimising NEC risk. A significant proportion of these growth retarded infants also have compromised blood flow to the gastrointestinal tract (GIT), potentially increasing their risk of developing NEC. It is, however, very important that SGA infants receive mainly breast milk for better tolerance and reducing the risk of NEC. Nutrition for SGA infants is equally vital after hospital discharge. Once SGA infants move away from the intrauterine and early post-natal negative influences on growth, their weight and height growth curves potentially cross percentile lines as they catch up on their genetic potential during the first 2 years of age. To facilitate this, post-discharge nutrition advice and monitoring are essential. The aim is to reach catch-up growth by the first 2 years to achieve weight and height > 10th percentile for age. To avoid the dangers of excessive catch-up growth, when weight velocity is greater than the average for post-natal age, the clinician must pursue a child's dietary history in detail.[121] In the National University Hospital, body mass index (BMI) charts are used for Singapore's pre-school children to detect undesirable weight gains.[122] About 10% of SGA infants nevertheless remain small at 2 years of age. These are the genetically small in whom growth hormone (GH) therapy is an option if the child's height remains < 2 standard deviations below the mean for age and sex at 3 years old. This option needs to be balanced between the potential gains in height versus the burden of prolonged treatment with GH.[123]

Overcoming nutrition-related growth failure

For the year 2013, 69.3% of the National University Hospital's VLBW infants were exclusively fed breast milk throughout their hospital stay, with the remainder fed breast milk supplemented with breast milk substitute feeds. Breast milk itself, however, has insufficient caloric and protein content for preventing post-natal growth failure in preterm infants. Breast milk content has been found to be highly variable. Its protein content decreases with time after birth.[124] Zachariassen et al. have studied the macronutrient contents in the milk from mothers who gave birth very prematurely, and investigated possible associations between macronutrients and certain maternal and neonatal characteristics.[125] Their results indicated that the content of protein in breast milk varies between mothers. It also reduces within weeks after a very preterm birth. Other factors associated with a lower protein content and higher fat and energy in the milk were previous breastfeeding experience and low gestational age, respectively. They commented that differences between individual breast milk composition could possibly influence nutrition and therefore bring about the need for an individualised approach when fortifying breast milk for preterm neonates.[125]

It is necessary that breast milk is supplemented with milk fortifiers for good post-natal growth.[105,125,126] Fortifiers are mostly bovine derivatives although those made from breast milk are now available in the US.[127] The various commercial fortifiers are fairly similar in content (see Appendix). They help to boost the protein and caloric content of breast milk and also supplement micronutrients like calcium, zinc, and multivitamins. The use of fortifiers has been found not to be associated with NEC.[128] Analysis of protein content of breast milk for an individual patient enables the clinician to selectively modify the amount of protein fortification. This is now practical with the introduction of bedside analysers.[129,130] There are also simple and relatively cheap analysers to measure creamatocrit (caloric content of breast milk) at home, which can help mothers to monitor the energy content of their expressed breast milk (EBM) supplied to their preterm infants (see also Chapter 3). As one Malaysian study found, storage of breast milk within a short period reassuringly does not significantly reduce its caloric content.[103] The use of bedside analysers routinely in the NICU, however, has not yet been subject to rigorous cost benefit reviews.

As nutritional composition of breast milk may be suboptimal despite fortifiers, an alternative approach is to add breast milk substitutes specialised for preterm (24 kcal/oz) to every other feed. Extra protein in the form of whey protein concentrate can be used to further boost the protein content in EBM. Some newer liquid formulations that are sterile and reportedly contain even higher protein are promising for better VLBW infant growth.[131,132] Medium chain triglycerides (MCTs) are readily available for extra calories and are usually well tolerated up to 3 ml/kg/day. With MCTs, however, there is the possibility of complications such as micro-aspiration from gastro-oesophageal reflux (GER) leading to lipoid pneumonia and an increase in fat mass instead of lean mass.

When breast milk is unavailable, clinicians can generally choose between breast milk substitute for term (20 kcal/oz) or preterm (24 kcal/oz) or donor breast milk (unavailable in Singapore). Breast milk substitute for preterm have higher calories but in trials that compared breast milk substitute for preterm with donor breast milk, the former was associated with an increased NEC incidence.[133] There is however, scant data comparing breast milk substitute for term infants with donor breast milk. Though donor breast milk is not conclusively protective of NEC,[134] a Cochrane review indicated an associated risk of NEC with formula feeding.[133] As such when breast milk feeding is not possible, it is the authors' practice to start on standard ready to feed (RTF) breast milk substitute (20 kcal/oz), and later to switch to breast milk substitute for preterm when more calories are needed for better growth. With a standardised feeding regimen, the incidence of NEC in the authors' practice between 2003-2013 for the VLBW cohort was low at 1.7%, compared to the Vermont-Oxford Network average of 5.3%.[135] Data from Singapore demonstrates the importance of standardising feeding protocol as well as a high usage of breast milk in minimising NEC.[136]

Non-nutritive factors and growth failure

Growth can be affected by various issues including non-nutritive factors such as the improper technique of breastfeeding, the inability of the infant to suck well or take in enough milk, frequent spills during feeds, the need for supplementary oxygen, occult infection, and a non thermo-neutral environment.

To ensure infants in the authors' practice receive mother's own milk, all mothers are referred to a lactation consultant when their infants are admitted to the NICU. Mothers are educated on how to maximise their milk flow and how to properly handle breast milk expressed at home, its storage and transfer to the hospital. Kangaroo mother care (KMC) was introduced in the centre since 2012 and this also possibly enhanced the availability of breast milk.[137] KMC is initiated for those who are stable clinically (less than 3 episodes of apnoea a day), even while on nasal prong continuous positive airway pressure (NP-CPAP). NP-CPAP, which has been used routinely since 1991, plays a big role in limiting CLD. It also reduces the effort needed for breathing.[138] The infants are kept on NP-CPAP until they are asymptomatic and achieve growth targets. In order to maintain a thermo-neutral environment and minimise heat loss, infants are nursed in incubators up to 1.7 kg. Non-nutritive sucking via breastfeeding or the use of pacifier is initiated generally at 32 weeks. Speech therapists are also involved in the care and the goal is to get infants off gavage feeding and onto ad-lib breastfeeding as soon as they can.

Monitoring the growth of the preterm infant

Although the weight of a preterm infant may be increasing, this may not mean that he is catching up to his true potential. There are no guidelines on how much and how fast catch-up should be, but an infant should be within 10–15% of the normal weight for his age. Failure to monitor growth well could result in the infant achieving a lower growth potential.

Assessment of growth in terms of daily weight, and weekly length and occipito-frontal circumference (OFC) should be undertaken. Growth targets should be clearly identified, and deviations from optimal growth patterns discussed at ward rounds daily. Reporting caloric intake should be a clinical routine, as important as the review of vital signs. Calculating protein intake and making up for the insufficiency is especially important during the transitional period from full total parenteral nutrition (TPN) to full enteral nutrition.[139] Biochemical assessments include monitoring serum sodium, potassium, blood urea nitrogen (BUN), and ferritin. Serum calcium, phosphate and alkaline phosphatase are performed twice weekly to monitor for rickets of prematurity. Liver function test is done periodically during TPN therapy for possible cholestasis. Several preventable conditions in the VLBW infant contribute to growth failure and affect future neurodevelopment. These include nosocomial sepsis, CLD and NEC. Monitoring closely for such morbidities are necessary in every NICU, and quality improvement initiatives should take place whenever appropriate. If growth falters (less than 70 g/kg/week), a detailed nutritional analysis is required to identify the underlying causes. One intervention includes increasing feed volumes up to 200 ml/kg/day as tolerated.

At hospital discharge, it is important to recognise infants whose weights are < 10th percentile and one must take heed of this growth failure as a clinical problem that needs to be addressed expediently, with well-informed parents as care partners. Post-discharge nutrition guidelines from the European Society of Paediatric Gastroenterology, Hepatology and Nutrition (ESPGHAN)[140] may be followed and adapted according to nutritional resources available locally (see also Chapter 6). Getting the parents involved, teaching them about the importance of growth and nutrition, and empowering them with the knowledge and skills in nutritional intervention may prevent this from spiralling to growth deprivation. When transitioning to home care, parents should be prepared for challenges, as the infant may have difficulty adapting to the new home environment. Mothers should be trained to enhance nutrition for their child by boosting breast milk production, maximising milk output, ensuring the proper technique of milk expression to prevent contamination, and some developmental care techniques such as KMC method for enhancing parent and child bonding.

Key points summary

- The time in the NICU during the convalescent phase is a critical period for monitoring and optimising the growth of preterm infants, as a substantial number of preterm infants develop growth failure upon discharge from the nursery.
- The growth of preterm infants, particularly those who are SGA, need a progressively aggressive nutritional intervention for catch-up growth to compensate for the usually more conservative and often necessarily more cautious approach in the initiation of enteral feeding.
- If the infant is on breast milk alone, fortification of breast milk especially to boost protein intake is necessary to ensure optimum growth is achieved.
- Individualising nutrition to the preterm infant may require analysis of breast milk and targeted fortification of breast milk to boost protein intake so as to ensure optimum growth in a select group of infants with growth failure.
- Non-nutritive factors such as improper technique of breastfeeding, infant not sucking well with excessive spilling during feeding, occult infection and non-thermal neutral environment should be considered as some of the possible underlying causes of the infant growth failure.
- Careful monitoring and overcoming growth failure with nutritional intervention while the infant is in the nursery may prevent continuing post-discharge growth failure and related poor neurodevelopmental outcome.
- Multidisciplinary involvement of lactational consultants, speech-language therapists and caregivers in feeding the growing preterm infant while in the NICU, and engaging the family in discharge planning and adaptation to the home are also important measures in preventing continuing growth failure.

Chapter 5

Strategies and challenges in feeding the preterm infant with intrauterine growth retardation

- Fook-Choe Cheah -

What is known on this topic?

- Compromised blood flow through the placenta during pregnancy can restrict nutrient delivery to the foetus, leading to intrauterine growth retardation (IUGR), and causing infants to be born as small for gestational age (SGA). 4% of infants in Asia are both SGA and preterm.[141]
- The risk of feeding intolerance and necrotising enterocolitis (NEC) are greater in the **preterm SGA** infants who are already nutritionally compromised.
- The delay in feeding may add to the continued growth failure in these infants.

What this chapter adds?

- Discusses the evidence and strategies in promoting early nutrition intervention for **preterm SGA** infants. Highlights special precautions for the very **preterm SGA** and extremely low birth weight (EBLW) infants who have greater risk of feeding intolerance and NEC even with a carefully monitored feeding regimen.
- Highlights the importance of using breast milk to reduce the risk of feeding intolerance and NEC in these infants.
- Discusses the use of prokinetics (erythromycin) in refractory feeding intolerance cases.

Introduction

A foetus fails to reach its potential growth when IUGR, that is the estimated foetal weight < 10th percentile and/or the abdominal circumference is less than the 5th–10th percentile, occurs.[142] At birth, an infant with a body weight below the 10th percentile for gestational age is considered SGA. The IUGR or SGA condition is associated with adverse perinatal outcomes. The **preterm SGA** infant not only faces an increased risk of NEC from prematurity, but also an associated functional immotility of the gut which often delays the establishment of enteral feeding. Consequently, these infants become even more growth retarded as a result of the failure to achieve optimal foetal accretion rates during the post-natal period while recovering from prematurity-related conditions. Thus, clinicians should strive to avoid delaying feeds in these infants, but recognise that feeding intolerance would be commonly encountered and be vigilant for early signs of NEC. Issues and strategies for feeding these infants are particularly relevant in Asia, as infants here are more likely to have lower mean birth weight than Caucasian infants.[143-145] 4% of infants in Asia are both SGA and preterm.[141] The incidence however, is variable and may not be clearly reported based on gestational ages. The author's analysis over the recent two years at his own centre showed that the rate of **preterm SGA** infants was in fact higher, reaching up to 34%. Another survey involving low- and middle-income countries found rates differing slightly within Asia itself, with South Asia and Southeast Asia having higher prevalence (3% respectively) compared to East Asia and West Asia (2% respectively).[146]

Feeding issues and challenges

Preterm SGA infants who are IUGR because of placental insufficiency may have re-distribution of blood concentrated to vital organs, limiting the circulation of blood to the abdominal viscera. This abnormal circulation can be detected when the infant is still a foetus through antenatal ultrasound and Doppler assessment of foetal blood flow. This condition may persist up to a week after birth,[147] which may pose as an impediment to tolerance of enteral feeding in addition to increasing the risk for NEC. Abnormal umbilical artery flow is an independent risk factor for early onset NEC in premature infants.[148] As the SGA infants with this antenatal umbilical Doppler abnormality have significantly more feeding intolerance than SGA infants with normal flow,[149] feeding should be introduced and advanced more cautiously for the former.

The compromised nutrient delivery in the IUGR foetus becomes a challenge and more complex depending on how severe the intrauterine growth impairment has been and the gestation at delivery. Intrauterine hypoxia and polycythaemia causing hyperviscosity may further complicate matters and interfere with the success of enteral feeding. **Preterm SGA** infants take longer than the appropriate for gestational age (AGA) preterm infants to achieve full enteral feeds.[150]

Unlike the healthy foetus, the growth-restricted foetus receives less glucose, lactate, ketone bodies, and amino acid, resulting in reduced total body fat and lean mass. Feeding these infants early would expectedly improve their energy balance, but clinicians are still unclear on what is the appropriate lower limit of glucose level that such neonates can safely tolerate based on physical maturity and the underlying growth restriction. Generally, a venous level of ≥ 2.6 mmol/l may be acceptable.[151] Although hypoglycaemia is commonly encountered among these infants, hyperglycaemia may also be a problem. In one prospective analysis, 32% of very low birth weight (VLBW) infants (< 1500 g) had glucose levels of more than 10 mmol/l for at least 10% of the time, and increasing prematurity and small size at birth were cited as contributing factors.[152] Adjusting the glucose delivery rate or glucose infusion rate (GIR) (see Chapter 1) may suffice as the first line intervention rather than resorting to insulin therapy as in most instances the glucose intolerance is often transient.

The importance of early enteral feeding

Growth restricted infants are at risk metabolically from substrate deficiency with reduced energy stores. This state of nutrition emergency is amplified in **preterm SGA** infants. As such, an aggressive nutritional intervention approach is necessary. Availing total parenteral nutrition (TPN) support is also vital in the initial phase.

Minimal enteral feeds (MEF) should commence from Day 1 with colostrum as the choice feed before transitioning to breast milk, which is preferably fortified, when about one-half total enteral feeds has been administered. Giving breast milk as enteral feeds is associated with a reduced risk of NEC, which is recognisably higher in SGA infants. In one study, proactive enteral feeding of moderately **preterm SGA** infants with breast milk starting with 100 ml/kg/day and advancing to 200 ml/kg/day by Day 4 was shown to significantly reduce the risk of hypoglycaemia. It was also well tolerated.[153]

Several large trials have shown that the early introduction of feeds resulted in more rapid achievement of full enteral feeding without an increased risk of NEC in **preterm SGA** infants even with abnormal umbilical artery blood flow on Doppler. This was not associated with significantly more feeding intolerance.[39]

- Furthermore, a Cochrane review showed no statistically significant risk of NEC in infants who were given early enteral feeds compared to those who had delayed feeding (more than 5–7 days after birth); and some of the trials in this review did include growth-restricted infants with evidence of abnormal umbilical artery flow.[34] One of these trials was a large study involving 404 preterm infants with abnormal antenatal Doppler studies, from 54 hospitals across the UK and Ireland.[37] This study found growth-restricted preterm infants to be able to achieve full enteral feeding faster when enteral feeds was introduced earlier. There also appears to be no increased risk of NEC with the early introduction. Table 2 illustrates Abnormal Doppler Enteral Prescription Trial (ADEPT)'s[39] feeding schedule.
- Another Cochrane review found no difference between a slower feed advancement (15–20 ml/kg/day) and a faster rate (30–35 ml/kg/day) in the risk of NEC among **preterm SGA** infants above 1000 g.[43] However, infants who had slow advancement took significantly longer to regain birth weight (reported median differences of 6 versus 2 days) and to establish full enteral feeding (5 versus 2 days) than the group with more rapid advancement.[43]
- The author's own study also revealed that infants who were given feeds early achieved full feeding by 5.5 days compared to 7.9 days in the delayed group.[33] This positive effect of an early stimulation of the gut suggests that stable premature SGA infants should be started on enteral feeding as soon as possible. Figure 11 illustrates the feeding schedule used in the author's study.

Table 2. Recommended feeding schedule from the ADEPT trial.[39]

Day of feeding	Volume of milk according to birth weight (ml/kg/HOUR)				
	< 600 g	600–749 g	750–999 g	1000–1249 g	≥ 1250 g
1	0.5	0.5	0.5	0.5	1.0
2	0.5	0.5	0.5	1.0	1.5
3	0.5	1.0	1.0	1.5	2.0
4	1.0	1.5	1.5	2.0	2.5
5	1.5	2.0	2.0	2.5	3.0
6	2.0	2.5	2.5	3.0	3.5
7	2.5	3.0	3.0	3.5	4.0–4.5
8	3.0	3.5	3.5	4.0–4.5	5.0–5.5
9	3.5	4.0	4.0–4.5	5.0–5.5	6.0–6.25
10	4.0	4.5–5.0	5.0–5.5	6.0–6.25	
11	4.5–5.0	5.5–6.0	6.0–6.25		
12	5.5–6.0	6.25			
13	6.25				
14	Increase as required				

Reprinted from BMC Paediatrics, Vol 9(63), Leaf A, et al., ADEPT - Abnormal Doppler Enteral Prescription Trial, 2009, with permission from BioMed Central.

Figure 11. Recommended early feeding schedule for preterm SGA infants based on the Universiti Kebangsaan Malaysia (UKM) Medical Centre trial.[33]

```
┌─────────────────────────────────────────────────────────────────┐
│         Eligible premature SGA infants (1000-1800 g) admitted to │
│              the neonatal intensive care unit (NICU)             │
└─────────────────────────────────────────────────────────────────┘
                                 ▼
┌─────────────────────────────────────────────────────────────────┐
│                             Early:                               │
│              Feeding started within 12 hours of life             │
└─────────────────────────────────────────────────────────────────┘
                                 ▼
┌─────────────────────────────────────────────────────────────────┐
│   Feeding started at Day 1 with increments (Day 2 onwards) as below: │
│                                                                  │
│                     Day 1: 10 ml/kg/day                          │
│                     Day 2: 20 ml/kg/day                          │
│                     Day 3: 25 ml/kg/day                          │
│                     Day 4: 30 ml/kg/day                          │
│   Day 5: 35 ml/kg/day (reach 120 ml/kg/day and to off intravenous fluid/TPN infusion) │
│   Day 6 and onwards: 35 ml/kg/day until reach total feeding of 180 ml/kg/day │
└─────────────────────────────────────────────────────────────────┘
```

Reprinted from poster presented at 19th Annual PSM Perinatal Congress 2012, Bakon FA, et al., Premature small for gestational age infants: early versus delayed feeding, with permission from Perinatal Society of Malaysia.

Precautions and strategies in feeding the preterm SGA infant

It is perhaps justifiable to highlight here that caution is to be exercised in feeding the extremely preterm infant (less than 29 weeks and < 1000 g at birth) with abnormal antenatal umbilical Doppler flow. These infants are slow to tolerate enteral feeding and have the highest risk of NEC. An analysis of this cohort of preterm infants who were also IUGR suggests a more conservative introduction of enteral feeding and slower advancement may be the preferred approach to avoid feeding intolerance and NEC.[154] An advancement of not more than 20–25 ml/kg/day feed is probably prudent for this highest risk group of infants.

In term infants who are SGA/IUGR, when full enteral feeds are established, it is essential to monitor the growth trajectory to avoid an excessive rapid "catch-up". Crossing multiple centiles in the early growth phase may put these infants at risk of metabolic syndrome in later life. It is unclear whether a similar approach is applicable in the **preterm SGA** infant.[155] The preterm infant underwent a shorter programming period of growth restriction in the intrauterine environment than the **term SGA**. Achieving a more rapid growth to overcome the growth restricted trajectory may be beneficial for improved neurocognitive gains when balanced against the risk of metabolic syndrome later. **Term SGA** infants catching up quickly in the first 12 months may not be conferred the same advantage in neurodevelopmental outcome as in the preterm, but their risk for obesity and hypertension in early childhood, and metabolic syndrome in adulthood is well documented.[155] Conversely, in **preterm SGA** infants, an increased need for protein and minerals for more rapid growth to stimulate intrauterine growth accretion and to achieve gains in better neurodevelopmental outcomes in my opinion, should orientate us to focus on optimising linear and head growth at least for the first 2 years of life. The use of breast milk with added high protein intake for lean body mass deposition and greater neurocognitive gains may thus be a reasonable approach to take within this period.

Nevertheless, how fast and what is the optimum target for a **preterm SGA** to catch up on growth is still inconclusive. We should however monitor growth so as not to exceed "catch-up" rate above the 90th percentile during these early years. While it is logical to target linear growth rather than ponderal weight gain with increased adiposity/fat deposition, we are currently unable to distinguish with certainty the small number of infants who may be genetically small from other growth retarded **preterm SGA** infants. Future advances may see a role for biomarkers in identifying mutations and insulin-like growth factor-binding protein (IGFBP) levels in cases that are genetically small who may benefit from less aggressive nutritional intervention.[156] Early therapy using hormonal modulation of growth may be the preferred approach in these instances.

Metoclopramide, a prokinetic may be used to improve feeding tolerance in preterm infants.[157] Another prokinetic, erythromycin may also be helpful, but a 2008 Cochrane review found insufficient evidence on its use and safety.[158] Practitioners are also reminded of the reported association between erythromycin and hypertrophic pyloric stenosis.[158] A more recent randomised controlled trial (RCT) however, concluded that erythromycin at a lower dosage may benefit the special group of preterm infants with feeding intolerance at a lower dosage.[159] Erythromycin is a motilin receptor agonist, and the dose for prokinetic action is lower (3–12 mg/kg/day)[158] than that used for antimicrobial purposes (50 mg/kg/day). It may also be prudent to use a lower dosage regimen in general and to resort to higher dosing (12.5 mg/kg/dose) only in the more premature infants and refractory cases.[159]

Key points summary

- The preterm IUGR infant faces increased risk of NEC as well as associated functional immotility of the gut which often delays the establishment of enteral feeding.
- The state of nutritional emergency is amplified in preterm infants who are also SGA. This issue is particularly relevant in Asia, which has a higher prevalence of these infants.
- Early aggressive nutritional intervention is still the hallmark approach with TPN therapy as the mainstay of support in the initial phase.
- Early introduction of feeds even from the first day with steady increments could result in a more rapid achievement of full enteral feeding without significantly increasing the risk of feeding intolerance and NEC.
- Extremely preterm infants who are SGA and < 1000 g birth weight may need a more cautious approach, with early feeding initiation as well as smaller volumes of feed increments (up to 20 ml/kg/day) is recommended.
- A rapid "catch-up" in the early growth phase within the first years may be acceptable to simulate intrauterine growth accretion rates and better neurocognitive gains in **preterm SGA** infants. In balancing the risk of metabolic syndrome in later life, emphasis should be placed on optimising linear and head growth with higher protein and minerals, and using primarily breast milk as the source of feeds.
- Breast milk plays an important role not only in modulating the growth trajectory so as not to be excessively rapid in crossing multiple centiles but also in reducing the risk of NEC and feeding intolerance in these infants.
- The use of prokinetics such as erythormycin may be considered in some **preterm SGA** infants who are faced with refractory feeding intolerance.

Chapter 6

Post-discharge feeding for long term growth and health

- Fook-Choe Cheah -

What is known on this topic?

- Post-natal growth failure occurs in a sizeable proportion of preterm infants and this may continue after hospital discharge.
- The positive impact of adequacy in feeding of the preterm infant after hospital discharge on neurocognitive outcomes requires close monitoring of nutrition and growth especially during the early period of infant brain development.

What this chapter adds?

- Emphasis on the fortification of breast milk or the use of post-discharge formulas (PDFs), may be necessary intervention to overcome post-discharge growth failure.
- Improved bone mineralisation with added nutrients such as calcium and phosphorus in fortifier or PDF may limit the incidence of reduced linear growth.
- Pragmatic strategies to successfully implement, manage, and monitor post-discharge feeding.
- Highlights the achievement of successful exclusive breastfeeding upon discharge of preterm infants as an important milestone. However, the monitoring for inappropriate growth in these infants with regular follow-up and addressing the malnutrition with early interventions is also vital.

Introduction

Aggressive early post-natal nutrition comprising total parenteral nutrition (TPN), followed by high caloric content enteral feeds through the fortification of breast milk or the use of nutrient enriched breast milk substitute, are strategies to limit growth failure in preterm infants until hospital discharge. But as the extrauterine environment is markedly different from the intrauterine environment, the current "standard" for post-natal nutrition of preterm infants fails to stimulate in utero human foetal growth rate in so much as up to 16–33% of preterm infants still sustained post-natal growth failure upon discharge.[160] As such, these infants may need follow-on additional nutrients to catch up on their growth, avert the risk of infections and for improved neurodevelopment outcomes even when discharged home.

Post-discharge nutrition and neurodevelopmental outcomes

The window for "catch-up" in the post-discharge growth-retarded infant is a golden opportunity for nutritional intervention through careful and regular monitoring on follow-up. It is vital that this "window of opportunity" is recognised and seized accordingly. If accomplished early, the risk of growth retardation continuing later in life can be limited. In human infants, this critical period are approximately the first year for the development of head circumference and the first three years for final height.[161] The appropriate and most current post-natal growth curves should be used to identify infants who are growth retarded (see Appendix 3). The available data, seen in Figure 12 show a sizeable population of infants had poor growth. The lower the gestation at birth, the more substantial the proportion that were affected.[162] This problem is anticipated to be more extensive in less developed countries.

Appropriate post-discharge nutritional intervention is therefore necessarily considered to address specific nutrient deficits to promote optimal growth and neurodevelopment without overfeeding. The study by Cooke et al. of preterm infants (and particularly males) fed a PDF for 6–12 months indicated enhanced growth.[163] Several studies have found that feeding nutrient-enriched breast milk substitutes increases infant weight, length and head circumference.[164,165]

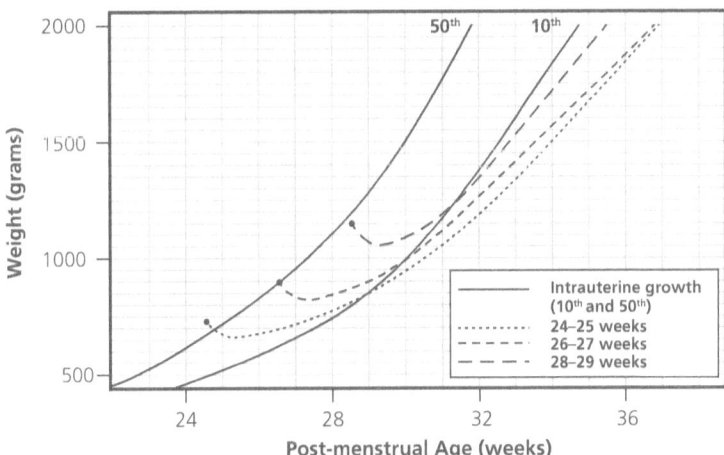

Figure 12. Average body weight versus post-menstrual age in weeks.[162]

Average body weight versus postmenstrual age in weeks for all study infants with gestational ages 24 to 25 weeks (dotted line), 26 to 27 weeks (short dashes), and 28 to 29 weeks (long dashes). The reference intrauterine growth curves were plotted using the smoothed 10th and 50th percentile birth weight data reported by Alexander et al.

Reproduced with permission from Pediatrics, Vol 104 No. 2, Page(s) 280-269, Copyright © 2009 by the American Association of Pediatrics.

Calcium-phosphate balance and linear growth

Preterm infants who have accumulated deficits in calcium and phosphorus by the time of discharge are at increased risk of poor bone mineralisation, metabolic bone disease, and reduced skeletal growth compared to term infants. The greatest risk for osteopenia occurs after discharge when there is rapid growth but the consumption of HMFs is usually discontinued.[166] The standard practice in many units is to give calcium 2.0 mmol/kg/day and phosphorus 0.5 mmol/kg/day as supplement or as human milk fortifiers (HMFs) in addition to breast milk until the infant attains a weight of 1800–2000 g. Some units may not practice post-discharge fortification wherein upon fully being breastfed at discharge it is deemed inappropriate to use the bottle to feed the fortified expressed breast milk. This may result in a proportion of infants after discharge who are at risk of poor bone mineralisation especially if calcium-phosphate supplementation was also neglected. The greatest at risk are all the extremely low birth weight (ELBW) and most VLBW infants. It is prudent to periodically check the bone profile of the infants with blood calcium, phosphate and alkaline phosphatase levels to intercept those that may have sub-clinical rickets for intervention. With therapy, reduced bone mineralisation in proportion to body weight gain generally improves. Bone mineralisation adjusted for anthropometric parameters in preterm infants reach values approximate to healthy term infants between 6 and 12 months of age and this seems to fit the skeletal and body size achieved.[167]

More rapid growth of preterm infants with improved nutrient intake was associated with improved neurocognitive outcomes.[113] However, in one study, there appears to be no neurodevelopmental advantage as infants fed with a nutrient-enriched breast milk substitute and standard breast milk substitute had similar Bayley mental developmental index (MDI) and psychomotor development index (PDI) scores at 18 months.[168] However, the numbers in this study were small and did not sufficiently represent infants of lower gestations.

Breast milk fortification and PDFs

After discharge, infants should optimally be breastfed. However, breast milk alone may be insufficient in many instances. This could be due to the lack of supply in mothers who have to return to work early. The threat of a substantial proportion with post-natal growth retardation and the high variability of nutrient composition in breast milk means that collectively, exclusive breastfeeding to post-discharge preterm infants may not be sufficient to meet the rapid growth of some infants. Although breast milk is preferred to breast milk substitute, supplementation with a PDF or breast milk fortification may be necessary under such circumstances for optimal growth. PDF have added nutrients especially calcium and phosphorus for improved bone mineralisation and is a logical supplement for mothers who are low in breast milk supply. According to the European Society of Paediatric Gastroenterology, Hepatology and Nutrition (ESPGHAN), infants discharged with a subnormal weight for post-conceptional age (PCA) who are fed on breast milk should be supplemented, for example with HMF, to provide adequate nutrient intake.[140] Feeding infants with unfortified breast milk was associated with slower ponderal and linear growths, higher risk of metabolic bone disease, and deficiencies in other micronutrients.[163]

In the author's practice, fortifying of breast milk is emphasised for the very preterm (< 30 weeks) extremely low birth weight (ELBW) infants as they have a higher risk of developing bone disease.[166] As HMFs are prescribed for inpatients, parents may opt to buy HMF or PDFs (or preterm breast milk substitute if PDFs are not readily available) as supplementation. With the breast milk substitutes, mothers with inadequate breast milk may alternate between breastfeeding and breast milk substitute feeding. Mothers who are fully breastfeeding are encouraged to fortify their expressed breast milk (EBM) for about 3-4 feeds daily. This is often acceptable and practical for mothers who are back to work when other caregivers administer the feeds over the usual 8-hour work period. PDFs are used in feeding non-breastfed preterm infants after discharge from hospital for a limited duration before they are reverted to term infant breast milk substitute. The PDF with higher contents of protein, minerals, and trace elements as well as long chain polyunsaturated fatty acids (LCPUFAs), ensures adequate growth at least until a PCA of 40 weeks, and possibly until about 52 weeks (3 months).[140] The growth-retarded preterm infant may benefit from the use of PDFs for even up to 9 months after hospital discharge. The Malaysian Paediatric Protocol states that specially formulated PDFs for preterm infants can be given to preterm infants with poor weight gain.[12]

In the author's practice, the average weight of preterm infants discharged from hospital was 1.8 kg at approximately 35-36 weeks corrected age. Commonly 30-50% of the EBM of the breast fed infant were fortified until 40-42 weeks corrected gestational age. The targeted groups are infants who are born < 32 weeks gestation or < 1500 g birth weight who fail to achieve appropriate weight gain for age despite receiving up to 200 ml/kg/day of breast milk. Infants not exclusively breast fed are given PDF as a supplement whilst those who are not on breast milk are given PDF as the sole feed. It is the author's opinion that infants born < 30 weeks gestation who are growing poorly (< 10th percentile of the growth curve), are the group most likely to benefit from PDF as an alternative to fortified breast milk. PDFs have a higher energy content of about 72 kcal/100 ml (22 kcal/oz) and at least 2 g/100 ml of protein (see Appendix 2). Once adequate growth velocity is established and growth measurements have reached the 25th to 50th percentile, the infant can be transitioned to breastfeeding exclusively or a standard breast milk substitute.

Monitoring and optimising post-discharge feeding

Preterm infants are to be monitored closely for feeding-related issues and growth, and are only discharged when firmly established on enteral feeding. After leaving the hospital, they may lose the benefit of constant monitoring to ensure they achieve the optimal growth potential. Even if these infants were deferred discharge, those who were born preterm had higher rates of morbidity than term infants.[169] Furthermore, logistical limitations may result in preterm infants being discharged earlier, especially in resource-limited countries, and inadequate follow-up or monitoring may contribute to delayed recognition and intervention of growth impediment. It is paramount that monitoring post-discharge feeding and growth is continued even after the infant leaves the hospital to seize the "window of opportunity" to intervene when growth is suboptimal.

Conversely, inadequate growth monitoring after discharge may also result in another potential complication of overfeeding. This is characteristically seen in the Asian context where mothers may be inclined or extended family members exert pressure to overfeed, especially the growth retarded or "small" infant.

Overfeeding is also most likely to occur during the catch-up growth period with the unregulated use of nutrient-enriched breast milk substitute. During this period, in an attempt to achieve post-natal weight gain as "equivalent" to intrauterine growth rate may potentially lead to a disproportionate increase in body fat.[170] This is particularly so if preterm breast milk substitute is used. The growth achieved with PDFs, however, is reportedly more resultant in an increase in lean body mass than an increase in fat.[171] If extrapolated to the preterm category, the greater risk of development of cardiovascular diseases and insulin resistance syndrome in later life particularly among the term small for gestational age (SGA) infants due to overfeeding and excessive catch-up[172] may be of concern. A targeted growth around the 25th–50th centile weight for age may be prudent when these long-term consequences of early nutrition are balanced against the potential neurocognitive gains in the shorter term.

Personal practice tips on post-discharge feeding of the preterm infant most at risk (< 30 weeks and/or < 1250 g) or with growth failure (< 10th percentile of weight)

- Preterm infants could benefit from PDF or HMF supplementation, especially if they are discharged home at weights lower than the 10th percentile of weight for age.
- There are no concrete guidelines on the amount and frequency of fortification, but fortifying about three feedings a day (HMF added to EBM) is practical. This frequency is pragmatic to fit into the mother's work schedule of 8–9 hours. After work or during weekends, exclusive breastfeeding can be resumed.
- Fathers can be involved in feeding the fortified EBM to the infant, allowing an opportunity to bond with their child, and giving mothers some respite.
- If HMFs are unavailable or limited in access, breastfeeding may be supplemented with preferably PDF or preterm breast milk substitute as alternative. Supplementing with PDF is also an option for mothers who have insufficient breast milk.
- Infants may be fed with fortified EBM or a PDF for up to 3 months term corrected age, and this may be continued if growth has still not caught up adequately. Monitor the growth of the infant closely to avoid excessive catch-up, preferably maintaining at 25th–50th percentile weight for age.
- PDFs should be stopped when the infant's gain in weight crosses centiles rapidly to the 75th–90th percentile. Infants could then revert to being breastfed exclusively or fed with a standard (term) breast milk substitute.

Key points summary

- At discharge, many of the VLBW and most ELBW preterm infants have subnormal weights; and with an unsupplemented diet, they may continue to have faltering growth.
- These infants, especially those who are SGA need higher amounts of nutrients compared to healthy appropriate for gestational age (AGA) preterm infants. This is especially problematic when they are discharged early, increasing their risks of not achieving their growth potential.
- Nutritional intervention should include breast milk fortification or PDFs to provide higher amounts of protein, energy, and minerals with HMFs until a satisfactory growth trajectory is reached.
- PDFs are preferred to term or preterm breast milk substitute for preterm infants at risk for growth retardation. Overfeeding, especially with the use of preterm breast milk substitute can result in excessive catch-up growth which is a precursor of obesity and its various associated long-term consequences. On the other hand, term breast milk substitute lacks in calories and extra minerals to support optimal growth.
- Close monitoring of post-discharge nutrition and growth is essential in the follow-up care of the high risk preterm infants.

Chapter 7

Prebiotics and probiotics: relevance and impact on preterm nutrition (in the Asian context)

- Girish Deshpande & Sanjay Patole -

What is known on this topic?

- The health benefits from probiotics and prebiotics in the prevention and treatment of various diseases are increasingly gaining evidence.
- The risk of necrotising enterocolitis (NEC), a major cause of mortality in preterm infants, is significantly reduced with the use of breast milk feed and antenatal glucocorticoids.
- Probiotics is an emerging and promising preventive therapy for NEC as shown in various randomised controlled trials (RCTs) and meta-analyses.

What this chapter adds?

- Summary of systematic reviews of 24 RCTs (24 trials, ~ 6000 neonates) showing that probiotics reduce the risk of death and definite NEC while facilitating milk feeding in preterm very low birth weight (VLBW) neonates.
- Emerging evidence for the role of probiotics in accelerating the establishment of enteral feeding in the preterm infant by reducing feeding intolerance and gastro-oesophageal reflux (GER).
- Exploring the evidence of prebiotics from RCTs indicates that prebiotics have a bifidogenic effect on the gut flora but their benefits on NEC is limited.
- Discussion of the logistics and benefits in implementing probiotic and prebiotic supplementation in preterm neonates with a focus in resource-poor settings and the Asian region.

Recently, there has been a significant interest in the field of probiotics and prebiotics for the prevention and treatment of various diseases. This chapter focuses on the benefits of probiotic and prebiotic supplementation in the preterm neonate.

Probiotics for preterm neonates

Definition: The United Nations Food and Agricultural Organisation and the World Health Organisation (WHO) define probiotics as "live microorganisms which when administered in adequate amounts confer a health benefit on the host".[173]

Probiotics for prevention of NEC in preterm neonates

NEC is the most common gastrointestinal (GI) surgical emergency in preterm neonates with potentially disastrous consequences.[174,175] An inappropriate excessive pro-inflammatory response by the immature innate immune system in response to stimulation by pathogenic bacteria in the gut is currently considered as the main reason for the development and progression of NEC in very preterm neonates.[176] Evidence also indicates the altered gut microbiome ("dysbiosis") as an important risk factor for NEC.[177]

The incidence of NEC has not changed significantly over the last 30 years despite the advances in neonatal intensive care. NEC continues to occur in 5–10% of VLBW neonates or in 1–2% of all nursery admissions. It is also one of the leading causes of death in preterm neonates who survive the first week of life.[174,175,178,179] The mortality related to definite (≥ Stage II) NEC is between 15–30% with higher rates seen in VLBW neonates (24–30%)[174,178] increasing to ~ 100% in those with full thickness widespread gut necrosis.

The morbidity of definite NEC is significant and includes prolonged hospitalisation, survival with short bowel syndrome, and long term neurodevelopmental impairment (NDI), especially in extremely low birth weight (ELBW) neonates needing surgery for the illness.[180-184] Schulzke et al. have systematically reviewed observational studies reporting long-term neurodevelopmental outcomes in VLBW neonates surviving after NEC. The risk of long-term NDI was significantly higher in the presence of at least Stage II NEC versus no NEC (Odds Ratio, OR: 1.82; 95% Confidence Interval, CI: 1.46–2.27). Patients requiring surgery for NEC were at higher risk for NDI versus those managed medically (OR: 1.99; 95% CI: 1.26–3.14). Results of analyses based on study design, follow-up rate, and year of birth were not statistically significantly different from those of the overall analysis. Risk of cerebral palsy and cognitive and severe visual impairment was significantly higher in neonates with NEC.[183] The economic burden of NEC is significant considering its complications that often prolong the hospital stay. Bisquera et al. have evaluated the impact of NEC on length of stay and hospital charges in a case-control study. The estimated total hospital charges for neonates with surgical NEC based on length of hospitalisation was USD $186,200 in excess of those for controls. Costs for medical NEC averaged in excess of USD $73,700 compared to controls. The excess hospital charges per year for NEC were USD $6.5 million or USD $216,666 per survivor.[185] Based on this data, the annual expenses towards NEC are estimated to be as high as 1 billion dollars per year in the USA, without accounting for the long-term care of survivors with NDI.

Current treatment for definite NEC is limited to bowel rest, and antibiotics. The additional options for Stage III NEC include peritoneal drain and/or surgery. Considering the significant burden of NEC, prevention is the only option. However the poorly understood pathophysiology of the illness has been the main reason for the difficulties in developing strategies for prevention of NEC. Current options are limited and include antenatal glucocorticoids, and early preferential feeding with breast milk.[186] However, the latter strategy is often defeated by the lack of mother's own milk and limited donor breast milk facilities.

Mechanisms of benefits of probiotics

Prophylactic probiotic supplementation is a promising new intervention for the prevention of NEC in preterm neonates.[177,187]

- **Appropriate gut colonisation:** It is well known that the preterm gut has low diversity of bacterial flora, and increased colonisation by pathogenic bacteria due to reasons such as delayed milk feeds, frequent exposure to antibiotics, and prolonged stay in the intensive care unit. Probiotic microorganisms improve the diversity of the gut microbiome, compete with pathogens for the epithelial binding sites, secrete antimicrobial peptides, and produce bacteriocins to actively inhibit the growth of other bacteria.[178,188]
- **Modulating Toll-like receptors (TLR) interactions:** Probiotics act via TLRs such as TLR 2 and TLR 4 to produce protective cytokines (e.g. interleukine 6, IL-6) which mediate cell regeneration and inhibit cell apoptosis.[189] Different probiotics appear to affect TLR expression in different ways.[190] Probiotics not only modulate immune function to improve anti-pathogen activity, but also mediate inflammatory responses to pathogens by increasing Th1 cytokine profiles resulting in increased anti-inflammatory cytokines and decreased inflammatory cytokines.[191]
- **Anti-inflammatory effects:** A significant part of gut defense is immunologically mediated and the gut has receptors, which trigger various responses. Several probiotic strains including *Lactobacillus reuteri* and *Bifidobacterium bifidum* have been shown to decrease pro-inflammatory cytokines (e.g. IL-6, IL-10, TNF-alpha) and activate the production of anti-inflammatory cytokines.[192,193]
- **Improvement of gut barrier function:** Investigators have hypothesised that a compromised gut barrier, defects in the production and/or composition of mucous or its properties allow bacteria to invade the gut and contribute to the pathogenesis of NEC.[194] Probiotics play a significant role in regulating the intestinal defense mechanisms and improve the integrity and function of the gut barrier. Animal studies have documented the role of probiotics in the secretion of mucous, secretory immunoglobulin A (Ig A), and other bioactive factors to reduce gut permeability.[192]
- **Other mechanisms:** Recently, it is proposed that immaturity of Paneth cell function contributes to the risk of NEC in preterm neonates.[195] Paneth cells play an important role in providing the antimicrobial peptide/chemical barrier and protect the gut epithelial surface from NEC.[196] Paneth cells are present in the intestine of the human foetus at relatively low levels and have an immature function. Probiotics like *Bifidobacterium bifidum* are known to modulate Paneth cell function, and secrete antimicrobial peptides that may help prevent NEC.[197]

Probiotics for preventing NEC in preterm neonates – current evidence

Systematic reviews of RCTs have confirmed the benefits of probiotics in preterm neonates.[198-200] Deshpande et al.[198] reported the first systematic review of RCTs evaluating efficacy and safety of any probiotic supplementation (started within first 10 days, duration: ≥ 7 days) in preventing ≥ Stage II NEC in preterm (gestation < 33 weeks) VLBW neonates. A total of 7/12 retrieved RCTs (N = 1393) were eligible for inclusion in the analysis. Meta-analysis using a fixed effects model (7 trials, N = 1393) estimated a lower risk of ≥ Stage II NEC (Risk Reduction, RR: 0.36; 95% Confidence Interval; CI: 0.20, 0.65) and all-cause mortality (RR: 0.47; 95% CI: 0.30, 0.73) in the probiotic group. The risk of blood culture positive late onset sepsis (LOS: 6 trials, N = 1355) did not differ significantly between groups (RR: 0.94; 95% CI: 0.74, 1.20). Overall the results indicated that in general, probiotics may significantly reduce the risk of ≥ Stage II NEC and all-cause mortality in preterm VLBW neonates while significantly shortening the time to full enteral feeds (TFEF). The updated meta-analysis by Deshpande et al. (11 trials, 2176 neonates) reconfirmed the benefits of probiotic supplementation in reducing NEC, mortality, and the time to full feeds.[199] The recently reported results of the Australian RCT (n = 1093) confirmed the benefits of probiotics in reducing the risk of NEC in the presence of a low baseline rate of the illness (4.4% versus 2.0%), and high breast milk feeding rates.[201] The current Cochrane review (24 trials, 5538 neonates) strongly recommends a change in practice in favour of routine probiotic supplementation in preterm neonates.[200]

Impact of probiotics on enteral nutrition in preterm neonates

Athalye-Jape et al. have recently reported the results of their systematic review assessing the evidence on effects of probiotics on enteral nutrition in preterm (gestation < 37 weeks) or low birth weight (birth weight < 2500 g) neonates.[202] The meta-analysis of 19 out of 25 studies included (n = 4527 out of 5895) using random effects model determined that the estimated TEEF was shorter in the probiotic group (mean difference: -1.54 days; 95% CI: -2.75, -0.32 days; p < 0.00001, I² = 93%). Other benefits included lower instances of feed intolerance, improved weight gain and growth velocity, less time to switch from orogastric to breast feeds, and increased post-prandial mesenteric flow. In addition, probiotic supplementation did not cause any adverse effects. They emphasised that additional research is necessary to assess the optimal dose, duration, and probiotic strain or strains used specifically for facilitating enteral nutrition in this population. Strains that will not only reduce the risk of NEC but also facilitate enteral nutrition in preterm neonates will be highly desirable. Considerations of the strain specific effects (e.g. *Lactobacillus reuteri* DSM 17938) in preterm neonates are important in this context.[203-207]

Indrio et al. have reported that in a RCT, infants with functional GER, L. reuteri DSM 17938 (1×10^8 colony forming units [cfu]/day) had reduced gastric distension and accelerated gastric emptying compared with the placebo.[203] In addition, L. reuteri seemed to reduce the frequency of regurgitation. Indrio et al. have evaluated the effects of prebiotic or probiotic added to a standard breast milk substitute on gastrointestinal (GI) motility in a RCT in 49 neonates.[204] A total of 17 neonates were exclusively breastfed; 32 were randomly assigned to prebiotic added breast milk substitute (0.8 g/dl of a mixture of short chain galacto-oligosaccharides (scGOS) and long chain fructo-oligosaccharides (lcFOS), ratio 9:1, n = 10), a probiotic added breast milk substitute (L. reuteri 1×10^8 cfu/day, n = 10), or a breast milk substitute with placebo (n = 12) for 30 days. After the study, the prebiotic, probiotic, and breast milk group neonates showed a higher percentage of slow wave propagation on electrogastrography and faster gastric half emptying time on ultrasound compared with the placebo group neonates. Indrio et al. have also investigated the effect of dietary supplementation with a probiotic on feeding tolerance and GI motility in healthy breast milk substitute-fed preterm Infants (n = 30).[205] Ten were exclusively breastfed, and the other 20 were randomly assigned in a double-blind manner to receive either L. reuteri ATCC 55730 (1×10^8 cfu/day) (from which the daughter strain DSM 17938 is derived)[208] or placebo for 30 days. Weight gains per day were similar for the three groups and no adverse events were recorded. Neonates receiving probiotic showed a significant decrease in regurgitation and average daily crying time, and an increased number of stools compared to the placebo group. Gastric emptying rate was significantly increased, and fasting antral area was significantly reduced in both the newborns receiving L. reuteri and breastfed newborns compared to placebo.

Routine use of probiotics in preterm neonates

It is important to note that countries such as Japan, Italy, Finland, and Columbia have been using probiotics routinely for preterm neonates for over a decade and have not reported any significant adverse effects.[209-212] Deshpande et al. reported significant reduction in the incidence of NEC after introduction of routine probiotic supplementation for preterm neonates (0.06%, n = 146 versus 5.5%, n = 142) in Australia.[213] They used Infloran 250 mg capsule, a combination of Lactobacillus acidophilus and Bifidobacterium bifidum, at a dose of 2×10^9 cfu/day starting with the first feed, and continuing until 34 weeks' corrected age. Janvier et al. (Montreal, Canada) have reported a significant reduction in NEC (from 9.8% to 5.4%, p < 0.02) with the introduction of routine probiotic supplementation in addition to a non-significant decrease in death (9.8% to 6.8%), and a significant reduction in the combined outcome of death or NEC (from 17% to 10.5%, p < 0.05).[214] Hartel et al. have recently reported outcomes after routine supplementation with Lactobacillus acidophilus/Bifidobacterium infantis in a cohort (n = 5351) of VLBW infants.[215] Within the 3 year observational period, centres were categorised based on their probiotic strategy as: (1) no prophylaxis (12 centres); (2) changing from non-user to user of probiotics during observational period (13 centres); and (3) use before starting observation (21 centres). Probiotic supplementation was associated with a reduced risk for NEC surgery (Group 1 versus Group 3: 4.2 versus 2.6%, p = 0.028; change of strategy: 6.2 versus 4.0%, p < 0.001), any abdominal surgery, and hospital mortality, and improved weight gain/day, but no effect on blood-culture confirmed sepsis. In a regression analysis, probiotics were protective for NEC surgery (OR: 0.58, 95% CI: 0.37–0.91; p = 0.017), any abdominal surgery (OR: 0.7, 95% CI: 0.51–0.95; p = 0.02), and abdominal surgery and/or death (OR: 0.43; 95% CI: 0.33–0.56; p < 0.001). However, the controversy about probiotics for preterm neonates is expected to continue considering the recently presented results of the multicentre trial from UK (Probiotics in Preterm Infants Study, PiPS; N = 1310). Supplementation with *Bifidobacterium breve* did not improve the incidence of NEC, late onset sepsis (LOS) or mortality in preterm infants < 31 weeks gestation.[216] The reasons for these findings can not be explored at the time of this publication as the data is available only as an abstract of the conference proceedings. It is however important to note that the addition of the data from PiPS trial does not change the results of the authors' updated meta-analysis (to be published elsewhere).

Probiotics for preterm neonates in resource limited settings

The issue of probiotics for preterm neonates in a resource limited setting is complex. The options involve either implementing probiotics based on the evidence from systematic reviews of RCTs knowing that the majority of the trials have been conducted in developed nations, or implementing only after confirming their efficacy and safety in a large definitive RCT in such a set up. Choosing the first option may not be correct from a purist point of view that probiotic effects are strain specific. However, selecting the second option is also not easy considering the difficulties in conducting high quality large multicentre trials in resource limited settings. The availability of probiotic strains that are appropriate for the given population is also an important issue. Access to proven safe and effective probiotics may be difficult in resource poor settings.[217] The barriers include regulatory hurdles, product costs and logistical difficulties associated with importing a product and maintaining cold chain, and difficulties in providing ongoing independent safety and quality control. Availability of local minimal dataset with details on NEC, all cause and NEC related mortality, suspected and blood culture proven LOS, type of feeds and time to start and reach full enteral feeds (TFEF: 150 ml/kg/day) is important to assess the impact after introducing routine probiotic supplementation in preterm neonates. Benefits of probiotics may not be as significant as reported in clinical trials without simple and proven strategies (e.g. antenatal steroids, early preferential use of maternal or donor breast milk, avoidance of breast milk substitute, standardised feeding protocols and avoiding undue prolonged exposure to antibiotics) in place. Neonatal demographic characteristics such as gestation and presence of intrauterine growth restriction are an important issue as they determine the risk of NEC, duration of probiotic supplementation, and the cost-benefit ratio in the context of limited resources. Many units may also face limited availability of breast milk, and cultural and religious beliefs may hamper preferential use of donor breast milk in such circumstances.

Knowledge of the pattern of gut colonisation in preterm neonates in the nursery is beneficial for optimal probiotic supplementation in any set up. Dutta et al. have recently reported abnormal intestinal colonisation patterns in the first week of life in VLBW neonates admitted to their level III neonatal intensive care unit (NICU) in India.[218] Meconium/stool specimens were obtained on Days 1, 3, 5 and 7 from 38 neonates. On Day 1, 45% had sterile guts, and by Day 3, all infants were colonised predominantly by *Escherichia coli, Klebsiella pneumoniae* and *Enterococcus fecalis*. Only one isolate had *Lactobacilli*, while *Bifidobacteria* was not detected during the study period. There was an association between breast milk substitute feeding and *E. coli* colonisation. Development and spread of antibiotic resistance, probiotic sepsis, and altered immune responses in the long run, are the potential adverse effects of probiotic supplementation in preterm neonates. Availability of killed or inactivated probiotic strains with clinically proven benefits may help in not only avoiding such adverse effects but also in avoiding the need to maintain the cold chain from the manufacturer to the field user. Awad et al. have compared the effect of oral killed (KP) versus living *Lactobacillus acidophilus* (LP) in reducing the incidence of LOS and NEC in neonates.[219] A total of 150 neonates admitted on Day 1 were enrolled in this double blind RCT. A total of 60 neonates received LP, 60 received KP, and 30 received placebo. Both LP and KP reduced the risk of NEC (absolute risk reduction 16%, 15%, respectively) and 18% for LOS (absolute risk reduction 18%) compared with placebo whilst the incidence of both did not differ significantly between neonates receiving LP versus KP. Those receiving KP showed significantly lower incidence of NEC compared to placebo. The incidence of LOS did not differ significantly between both groups. There was significant reduction in LOS and NEC among those colonised with *Lactobacillus* compared to those not colonised at Day 7 (27.9 versus 85.9%, 0 versus 7.8%) and at Day 14 (48.7 versus 91.7% for LOS and 0 versus 20.8% for NEC). Given the global implications of these results, the benefits of inactivated/killed probiotics need to be assessed in further large definitive trials. Results of systematic reviews of RCTs indicate that probiotics do not reduce the risk of LOS.[199,200,220-222] It is however important to note that majority of these trials have been conducted in developed nations where *coagulase negative staphylococci* (CONS) are the predominant organism responsible for LOS. Though limited, the evidence from RCTs from resource limited setting indicates that probiotics may significantly reduce non-CONS related LOS.[223-225]

Human milk oligosaccharides (HMOs) and prebiotics in preterm neonates

Several bioactive agents in breast milk play an important role in infant protection and guide the growth and development of the GI tract and the brain.[225-227] Prebiotics are dietary ingredients, usually oligosaccharides (OS) that provide a health benefit to the host, mediated by the modulation of the human gut microbiota.[228,229] Breast milk has high levels of complex OS that influence the composition of the intestinal microbiota in breastfed infants.[230] Discovered more than 60 years ago, these HMOs, a family of structurally diverse unconjugated glycans, constitute the third most abundant class of molecules in breast milk.[91,231-235] The concentration of HMO reaches up to 20 g/l in early breast milk.[234] HMOs comprise close to 200 structures[228] and are known to facilitate growth and development of the intestine and its immune system, and microbial ecosystem flora.[236-239] The impact of three predominant HMOs on multiple aspects of enterocyte maturation in vitro were assessed by Holscher et al.[236] Their results suggest differential roles for specific HMOs in maturation of the GI tract. The structure of HMO and its connection to bacterial and intestinal epithelial cells' digestibility, membrane transportation and catabolic activity is vital in determining the composition of intestinal microbiota.[240]

HMOs were discovered initially as a prebiotic "bifidus factor" to provide health benefits in breastfed neonates as it could be used as a metabolic substrate for desired bacteria and shaping the intestinal microbiota composition.[91] They are anti-adhesive antimicrobials that serve as soluble decoy receptors, prevent pathogen attachment to infant mucosal surfaces and lower the risk for viral, bacterial, and protozoan parasite infections.[237,241-243] In addition, HMOs may modulate epithelial and immune cell responses, reduce excessive mucosal leukocyte infiltration and activation, lower the risk for NEC and provide the infant with sialic acid as a potentially essential nutrient for brain development and cognition.[91,244] Jantscher-Krenn et al. have reported that HMO reduced NEC in neonatal breast milk substitute-fed rats and the effects were highly structure specific.[245] Their results indicate the potential of disialyllacto-N-tetraose (DSLNT) to prevent or treat NEC in breast milk substitute-fed infants. In addition, its concentration in the mother's milk could serve as a biomarker to identify breastfed infants at risk of developing NEC.[245]

The metabolism of HMO is complex. Unlike major breast milk nutrients such as lactose, lipids and proteins that are easily digested and assimilated by infants, certain molecules such as HMO and glycosylated proteins and certain lipids tend to evade intestinal digestion and move through the GI tract.[246] By preventing the colonisation of enteric pathogens and providing carbon and nitrogen sources for other commensals in the colon, the HMOs influence the composition of the developing intestinal microbiota in the infant.[246] *Bifidobacterium* species of bacteria probably contribute their predominance as intestinal microbiota in the first year of life as they are one of the very few bacteria that gains access to the energetic content of milk. These bacteria utilise HMOs and target other breast milk glycoconjugates.[246]

The OS that are added to infant breast milk substitute differ from naturally occurring HMOs structurally, making them unable to provide some of the structure specific effect.[226] The common mixture of prebiotics contains scGOS/lcFOS, (ratio of 9:1) to closely resemble the molecular size composition of HMOs.[247] Effects on stool consistency and frequency have been observed in many studies in healthy term and preterm infants using breast milk substitutes containing scGOS/lcFOS (ratio 9:1). This effect on stool consistency indicates that scGOS/lcFOS may have a role in reducing the risk of constipation.[247] The mixture of scGOS/lcFOS induces an increase in *Bifidobacteria*, similar to that of breastfed infants.[239] The resulting changes from its ingestion include high concentrations of lactate, a slightly acidic pH, and high acetate and low butyrate and propionate levels.[248]

HMO composition varies between mothers and throughout lactation. Marx *et al.* have compared the HMO content between donor breast milk with mother's own milk.[234] Their results showed that compared to human milk, donor milk HMO amount, concentrations of lacto-N-tetraose, lacto-N-neotetraose, lacto-N-fucopentaose 1, and disialyllacto-N-tetraose were significantly lower whereas the concentrations of 3'-sialyllactose and 3-fucosyllactose were significantly higher. They concluded that infants receiving donor milk are likely to ingest HMO at different total amounts and relative composition from what they would receive with their mother's own milk. The need for studies assessing the importance of a mother-infant match with regard to HMO composition was pointed out.

In a study to determine the influence of specific HMO on the growth and metabolic products of human intestinal microbiota, Yu et al. fed each of the 25 major intestinal microbiota isolates with individual major fucosylated and sialylated HMOs in an anaerobic culture. Though specific *Bifidobacteria* and *Bacteroids* digested specific HMOs differentially, the major fucosylated HMOs stimulated key species of the beneficial microorganisms (mutualist symbionts). This suggests strategies that can be used to treating dysbiosis and associated inflammatory disorders.[249]

Based on their chemical structures, HMOs are divided into core-oligosaccharides, sialo-OS, fucosyl-OS, and sialo-fucosyl-OS. As glycosyltransferases enzymes are partially regulated by genetic mechanisms (expression of secretory and Lewis' genes), breast milk can be categorised into four different secretory groups.[90]

Clinical trials of prebiotic OS supplementation in preterm and term neonates

Srinivasjois et al. have conducted a systematic review of RCTs evaluating the safety and efficacy of prebiotic OS supplementation in preterm (gestation ≤ 37 weeks) neonates.[250] A total of seven trials (n = 417) were included in their review. Five trials (n = 345) reported the incidence of NEC, and three trials (n = 295) reported the incidence of LOS. Meta-analysis revealed no significant reduction with prebiotic use: a pooled relative risk (RR) and 95% CI as 1.24 (0.56–2.72) for NEC, and 0.81 (0.57–1.15) for the risk of LOS respectively. There was no improvement in time to enteral feeds post-intervention in three individual trials (n = 295). Meta-analysis indicated a statistically significant difference in the growth of *bifidobacteria* in the OS group (Weighted mean difference, WMD: 0.53; 95% CI: 0.33, 0.73 x 10^6 colonies/g, p < 0.00001). Reductions in stool viscosity and pH were also observed. There were no significant adverse effects related to the supplement in any of the trials.[250] Niele et al. have recently reported that there is no decrease in the incidence of allergic and infectious disease during the first year of life when preterm infants are supplemented with short-term enteral supplementation of non-human neutral and acidic OS during the neonatal period.[251] Rao et al. systematically reviewed RCTs on the efficacy and safety of prebiotic supplementation in full-term neonates.[252] A total of 11 of 24 identified trials (n = 1459) comparing breast milk substitute supplemented with or without prebiotics, commenced at or before the age of 28 days and continued for 2 weeks or longer were eligible for inclusion in their review. A significant increase (six trials) and a trend showing an increase (two trials) of bifidobacteria counts was seen after supplementation. The estimated significant reduction in stool pH in infants who received supplementation was determined by a meta-analysis (WMD: -0.65; 95% CI: -0.76 to -0.54; six trials). Compared with the controls, the supplemented neonates had marginally better weight gain (WMD: 1.07 g; 95% CI: 0.14–1.99; four trials) with softer and frequent stools similar to breastfed infants. All except one trial reported that prebiotic supplementation was well tolerated. In that trial, parents of infants given prebiotic supplementation reported diarrhoea (18% versus 4%; p = 0.008), irritability (16% versus 4%; p = 0.03), and eczema (18% versus 7%; p = 0.046) more frequently. Results of a systematic review of RCTs indicated that a prebiotic OS supplement added to term infant feeds may prevent eczema.[253] However, it is unclear whether the supplementation should be restricted to infants at high risk of allergy or whether it may have an effect on low risk populations; or other allergic diseases including asthma.[253,254] Further studies are needed to assess whether early prebiotic and probiotic supplementation may alleviate symptoms associated with crying and fussing in preterm infants and colic in term infants.[254,255] Evidence from current clinical trials does not indicate a protective benefit from prebiotic supplementation on the rates of NEC and LOS.

Key points summary

- Current evidence suggests that probiotics offer significant benefits in terms of prevention of NEC, mortality, and establishing enteral nutrition in preterm neonates.
- Further research is necessary before high quality safe and effective probiotics for preterm neonates, are implemented in resource-poor settings.
- Inactivated/killed probiotics may be an attractive option in resource-poor settings but further research is required to confirm their safety and efficacy.
- A consistently decreased risk of NEC in trials using different probiotic strains and protocols suggests a non-strain specific protection.[256]
- Prebiotic OS supplementation appears to be safe and effective in promoting a gut microbiota that is closer to that in healthy breastfed term infants. However, there is insufficient evidence that prebiotic OS may protect against NEC or LOS.
- Conducting large and definitive RCTs assessing clinically important outcomes related to prebiotic OS supplementation alone in the neonatal period,[250] may be more appropriate in countries which cannot adopt probiotic supplementation as a standard of care for various reasons.

Chapter 8

Cultural beliefs and practices influencing breastfeeding of the preterm infant
- *A survey of reported experiences from neonatologists in the Asian region*

- Fook-Choe Cheah -

What is known on this topic?

- Not much is known but evidence suggests breastfeeding rates may be influenced by social and economic factors.
- The Asian region is ethnographically diverse with variation in social-cultural practices, beliefs and religions sufficiently deep-rooted to influence breastfeeding practices among mothers of preterm infants.

What this chapter adds?

- Results from a survey of personal experiences of neonatologists from their encounter with mothers breastfeeding their preterm infants in this region.
- The results highlighted some important factors based on cultural beliefs that may influence the process of breastfeeding the preterm infant.
- It is hoped that results of this survey could spur future studies to explore how some of the more commonly encountered factors may impact the rate of breastfeeding in this region.

Introduction

The beneficial effects of breastfeeding are well established and increased awareness is further promoted by the World Health Organisation (WHO) Baby-Friendly Hospital Initiative commencing in 2002. It strongly recommends the need for exclusive breastfeeding from birth to 6 months, and continued breastfeeding for at least two years with timely and appropriate introduction of complementary feeding.[257] Breastfeeding rates across the world still differ greatly and this may be attributed to various factors such as logistics in providing support facilities, educational awareness, cultural practices during the confinement period and even the overall perception of the society.

WHO's compilation of data from 21 European countries revealed a wide disparity in the initiation of breastfeeding for infants in that region. Only nine of the countries had more than 50% rate of early initiation of breastfeeding within 1 hour after birth.[258] Scandinavian countries particularly have shown high rates due to their family-centred care model, with couples having the option to accompany their infant round-the-clock in the neonatal intensive care unit (NICU), as well as prevalent lactation support and counselling. In Sweden, 98% of all infants included in a population survey received breast milk within the first week of life.[259] Most Scandinavian countries also have high employment rates and low income inequality, and offer various benefits for parents which include fully salaried time off work with extensive pre- and post-partum support.

Breastfeeding patterns in Asia also varied significantly. In Indonesia, 66% of the infants were breastfed within 1 day of life[260] and timely initiation of breastfeeding occurred in 63.7% of infants in Malaysia.[261] About half of the infants (57%) in Bangladesh are breastfed within the first hour.[262] In Pakistan, only 18% of infants received breast milk within 1 hour of birth and slightly more than half (58%) within 1 day of life.[263] Almost all infants (96%) included in a National Survey in Singapore were being breastfed at discharge.[264] One survey conducted in four public hospitals in Hong Kong revealed that less than one third of the mothers breastfed their infants within the first hour of birth and this figure fell to less than 20% when determining the number of infants who were exclusively breastfed while in hospital.[265]

Contrastingly breastfeeding rates and practices involving specifically preterm infants are rarely documented. In this chapter, a survey of a select group of neonatologists in Asia reported on some of the maternal beliefs, perceptions and socio-cultural practices as well as logistic issues that may affect breastfeeding of preterm infants in their settings. Their responses were compiled in a survey which also addressed unit practices or protocols for breastfeeding and handling of breast milk. Twenty one neonatologists from six countries responded to this survey (Indonesia = 8, India = 4, Malaysia = 3, Singapore = 3, Hong Kong = 2, and Thailand = 1). The respondents were primarily from the major public and private hospitals in capital cities.

Maternal beliefs and perceptions of breastfeeding preterm infants in Asia

Mother's ability to breastfeed

In the survey, 33% of neonatologists encountered mothers claiming that breastfeeding is a strenuous activity and that they were physically weak to breastfeed during confinement. The confinement period is at least for one month and can last for six weeks. They also found mothers frequently claiming to be unwell to breastfeed because of simple cough and cold illnesses. These perceptions have been reported elsewhere[266] and can be overcome with proper education during lactational support counselling.[267] For mothers to successfully breastfeed their infants, lactation support should be initiated preferably even before delivery. As delivery of infants in preterm births are often unexpected, the mother is left unprepared, thus impeding successful breastfeeding. Perhaps hospitals should start initiating ante-partum classes early, so that mothers start enrolling for these even from the time they conceive. These classes should not only provide information on the benefits of breastfeeding, but also on proper breastfeeding techniques and addressing common problems with breastfeeding.[268] In Singapore, a breastfeeding hotline was set up to help with lactation. Similarly, a study in Malaysia found that telephone counselling offered by nurses who have been certified as lactation counsellors improved breastfeeding rates at 1 month after delivery.[269] This could partly address the problem of inadequate staffing that limit direct contact between nurses and mothers. Culturally, mothers in the Malay communities in Malaysia and in Indonesia commonly practise post-partum massage (known locally as *urut*) to improve their physical health and strength, which may also help them to lactate. One study in Indonesia, also reported the beneficial effects of *Saoropus androgynous* (locally known as *katuk* leaves), which is commonly ingested by breastfeeding mothers in the community to improve lactation. Starting breastfeeding within 1 hour of delivery also positively affects breastfeeding success.[270]

It was reassuring that more than 95% of the neonatologists surveyed reported that mothers did not feel that breastfeeding delayed physical recovery after delivery or inhibited their recuperation process during confinement, predisposed to chronic illness in later life/old age, prevented them from maintaining a slim figure or hampered weight reduction. The majority also did not feel that breastfeeding would affect their relationship with their husband. However, about one-fifth of the surveyed neonatologists reported some mothers actually believed breastfeeding would cause breast disfigurement or size disproportion. This misconception should be dispelled in post-partum classes or during clinic follow-up.

A majority of the neonatologists (80%) also encountered mothers having the perception that small breast sizes were not able to produce sufficient milk, and all have met with mothers who frequently complained that their infants were probably not getting enough milk or that milk was deemed not flowing sufficiently well. This had been reported elsewhere.[271] This is often one of the predisposing factors that cause mothers to supplement feeds with breast milk substitutes once the preterm infant is discharged home. However, the issue of whether infants are getting enough milk from breastfeeding may not invoke the same anxiety when their preterm infants are cared for in the hospital as they are visibly fed with the specified amounts of expressed breast milk (EBM) when not directly breastfed. As such, before the infants are discharged home mothers should be encouraged to room-in and learn from experience the signs of infant satiety when directly breastfed. During this time, mothers should also be educated that the initial transient drop in weight experienced by the infant is acceptable and not due to insufficient milk supply. Positive reinforcement can be offered to highly sceptical mothers by educating them about the expected volume of feeds for their infant and allowing the mothers to witness for themselves the amount expressed that will meet this requirement. Aside from recognising infant satiety, the usual duration taken for an adequate feeding episode, interval between feeds and breast "empty-feel" after each successful feed may also be conveyed during this process. The expected average in normal infant weight gain can also be instructed for their own periodic self-monitoring at home and reassurance. Mothers should also be taught how to add fortifiers to the EBM for their preterm infant if necessary.

Bonding and infant-related factors

Another frequently reported encounter was the infant refusing to suck on the breast. This may occur in cases with insufficient rooming-in opportunities resulting in maternal lack of confidence in breastfeeding. Mothers need to be reassured that as preterm infants are often initially tube-fed, they are likely to have some oral aversion to sucking on the breast and also problems with swallowing coordination, making the transition to breastfeeding challenging at times. These impediments could be addressed if hospitals provide generous rooming-in facilities to enable mother and child to bond and establish breastfeeding together, as well as engage speech therapists to help infants by stimulating the maturation of their sucking and swallowing motions.

Factors relating to the lactating mother's diet and medications

It is encouraging to note that 80% of the neonatologists dealt with mothers who did not avoid eating nutritious foods or were restricted in their dietary intake during the lactation period. Some communities in Asia, particularly in the rural areas reportedly restrict fluid intake as part of the traditional post-partum rituals in the confinement period.[272] Although not a prevalent issue, it is still disconcerting that 10% of practitioners had encountered this among their patients. The importance of adequate fluid intake during breastfeeding should be emphasised by re-educating mothers who may practise this restriction.

Another common problem is mothers ceasing breastfeeding because of their intake of prescribed medications, as all of the neonatologists have encountered this, with 38% having to deal with it frequently. Mothers cited fear of harming their infant from transferred medications in their breast milk. Addressing this in post-partum classes and having a pharmacist relay the pertinent accurate information while counselling mothers on medication use during pregnancy is advantageous to allay the fears that may impede breastfeeding. Directing mothers to valuable online resources on medications and chemicals that breastfeeding mothers can be exposed to, such as the online database of the US National Institutes of Health LactMed® (Available at http://toxnet.nlm.nih.gov/cgi-bin/sis/htmlgen?LACTMED) may be of use.

On the other hand, ingesting traditional medicines/supplements perceived to be good for her health did not appear to be a cited reason for cessation of breastfeeding. Although suspect, we have limited data to date as to which of these traditional herbs may impact breastfeeding significantly.

Breast milk and breast milk substitutes

A survey conducted during the mid-1980s in Peninsular Malaysia revealed that educated, high income women living in urban areas were less likely to breastfeed or only breastfed for a short period, as they preferred to bottle feed.[273] This trend, however, is changing, partly due to WHO's aggressive promotion of breastfeeding in the latter years. Following on this, more than 85% of the surveyed neonatologists reported that generally mothers did not consider breast milk substitutes such as goat milk or soy milk to be superior to breast milk, nor did mothers consider the benefits of breast milk to be over-rated. Although the prevalent knowledge on the merits of breast milk is reassuring, many mothers are still unaware of the importance of colostrum and perceived it was too little to be useful, although they did not consider colostrum negatively as "dirty breast discharge". A review of the literature in the 1990s revealed that colostrum was normally discarded among Asian communities.[274]

Three quarters of the neonatologists reported that mothers were involved in sharing their breast milk, and this was commonly encountered in Malaysia and Indonesia. This was likely influenced by ethnic and religious beliefs, as the population in these countries are predominantly of the Muslim faith that may allow "one-to-one" donor milk sharing when donor milk banks are not feasible. Donor human milk banks where pooled breast milk is processed is not religiously acceptable to Muslims as opposed to "one-to-one" sharing when both donor and recipient consent to the process and are prepared to face the related health and legal implications.[89] These conditions should be explored positively and expanded pragmatically in countries citing similar religious hurdles in using donor milk when mother's own milk is not available.

Logistics

One of the major factors impeding the continuation of breastfeeding is having to return to a regular job or working life. This has been reported in numerous studies which cite work commitments as one of the reasons for non-exclusive breastfeeding or stopping breastfeeding early.[266,271,275-277] Another logistic issue, which is particularly relevant in the context of the preterm infant is the difficulty for mothers who are still in confinement to travel to the hospital to breastfeed their infants. In Asian communities, mothers are normally restricted from leaving the house during the confinement period. For those who do not have this restriction, their visits to the hospital may be limited because of the lack of transportation and most would depend on their husbands to facilitate this. Lack of child-care support also means that many remain at home to care for their other children. Family-centred care with rooming-in facilities modelled after the practices in Scandinavian countries or financial assistance for travel allowances and accommodation arrangements for the family as practised in some countries e.g. New Zealand, may help to alleviate this problem.

In Indonesia, there have been reports of courier service enterprises offering to transport expressed breast milk from the mother's home or office to the hospital, thus helping to ensure that infants in the hospital are regularly receiving their mother's own milk. Nevertheless, it should be cautioned that such service may not be adequately regulated and monitored for quality and safety of the transported EBM. As quality control is not guaranteed, issues such as inadequate cold storage and errors in delivery could arise.

Social influence

In this survey, the neonatologists also concurred that in the Asian setting the extended family does play a major role in the care of the mother after birth and her baby. As such breastfeeding can be affected due to family interventions and existing customs. Practitioners should consider this aspect by also counselling and educating the hierarchical figures in the extended family if necessary in order to achieve a positive impact towards success in breastfeeding.

Commentary on neonatologists' accounts and concerns with mothers handling of expressed breast milk

The majority of the surveyed neonatologists (95%) rarely or never encountered mothers who avoided breastfeeding or expressing breast milk because they were restricted from bathing, a confinement practice for some. This however, raises concerns with contamination of EBM from potentially heavy bacterial colonisation of the unwashed maternal skin. Also of concern is that many mothers did not practise adequate hand hygiene before expressing breast milk (as 80% of physicians have encountered this problem). In a Hong Kong study that looked into bacterial contamination of breast milk from mothers of very low birth weight (VLBW) infants, approximately two thirds had significantly high rates of bacterial contamination even with *Gram-negative bacilli*. The tradition of bathing avoidance after childbirth was implicated.[76] A Malaysian study also revealed that a majority of samples of breast milk expressed at home were culture positive.[78]

Most of the respondents rarely or never had parents complaining about the lack of storage facilities such as refrigerator or freezer to keep EBM for later use. Although most families boil milk bottles before use, one-third of neonatologists reported that they commonly encountered mothers who rinse bottles with water only. Majority of mothers reportedly re-use bottles whilst only some use disposable containers. Families that re-use bottles may limit the volumes of breast milk actually delivered to the hospital for their babies' consumption. Parents also find it inconvenient to have to frequently clean these containers especially if the boiling method is used to sterilise. Such time constraints may lead to short-cuts and non-compliance to sterility/adequate hygiene. Perhaps cheap disposable containers such as Bisphenol A (BPA)-free plastic bags can be a preferred, more viable option in such circumstances.

Although confronting with possible contamination, more than half of the neonatologists surveyed do not routinely culture EBM and do not commonly pasteurise breast milk obtained from mothers before being fed to their preterm infants. Pasteurisation may affect immune and bioactive components in breast milk,[79] potentially reducing its benefits. In Malaysia, some units do pasteurise EBM because of concerns of heavy bacterial contamination.[76] There is currently insufficient evidence to link either the type or load of bacterial contamination that increases the risk of necrotising enterocolitis (NEC) or infections to the preterm infant. As a precautionary measure however, routine surveillance may be necessary if there are high incidences of heavy bacterial contamination of EBM. Furthermore, regular surveillance may uncover sources of breast milk contamination that could be associated with outbreaks of NEC in some units, although some may debate the cost-effectiveness of such a measure. Pasteurisation in these instances may be a prudent interim measure in reducing or interrupting the outbreak. Pasteurisation is also useful to reduce the risk of transmission of bacteria and viruses in instances when donor milk is used especially in "one-to-one" sharing when the donor has not been previously screened.

The state of support services for lactating mothers and breastfeeding of preterm infants in this region

In this survey, a majority of the respondents (95%) reported having lactation consultants and some other forms of support services. In many settings, lactation consultants are part of the nursing staff who offer support during working hours. Some settings do utilise dedicated nurses to help support and advise mothers. In Singapore, there are lactation clinics run by nurses, midwives, and counsellors. In a Malaysian hospital, lactation consultants are outsourced to conduct home visits. In hospitals that do not have enough full-time lactation consultants, often nurses trained to provide lactation support undertake this responsibility. However, these nurses are often burdened with other work responsibilities leading to insufficient time expended to support or counsel mothers on lactation proper. Under-staffing and limited facilities that are only available during office hours may collectively pose a challenge to the success rate of breastfeeding of the preterm infant.

Majority of the respondents (90%) enforce the practice of kangaroo mother care (KMC) for the stable and growing preterm infants who are on full enteral feeding before they are discharged from the nursery. Although some settings would initiate KMC for a stable infant irrespective of gestational age or weight, most will not start for infants younger than 27 weeks gestation. Other limitations cited by the neonatologists were the lack of space and privacy. One neonatologist commented that the inability of the mother to be in the hospital for more than 3–4 hours a day makes extended KMC not possible. A neonatologist from Thailand shared that her hospital was the only setting in the country with full family-centred care that provides mothers with a room for overnight stay in the NICU. This allows mothers to be involved in the developmental care of infant virtually round the clock. Here mothers are encouraged to exclusively breastfeed as well.

Peer counselling has been found to be useful,[278] and most NICUs in this region have some form of support group for parents or breastfeeding mothers. In Indonesia, the breastfeeding mothers' association (*Kelompok Ibu Pendukung ASI*) have numerous innovative activities such as in engaging celebrities to encourage members to breastfeed. In Singapore, besides a breastfeeding mothers' support group, there is also a breastfeeding telephone hotline.

Key points summary

- Breastfeeding being perceived as a strenuous activity to postpartum mothers, insufficient milk and the inability of the infant to suck on the breast are some of the commonly reported misconceptions encountered in this region that impedes successful breastfeeding of the preterm infant.
- Logistic issues deterring mothers from breastfeeding include having to return to her full time job and the difficulty to travel to the hospital because of cultural restrictions in the post-partum confinement period, the lack of transportation or the need to care for other children at home.
- "One-to-one" sharing of donor breast milk may be an option for mothers who are unable to produce breast milk sufficiently especially in Muslim communities that generally do not accept pooled unknown donor milk such as the practice in donor milk banks. A standard processing procedure with clear guidelines on mutual acceptance and adequate monitoring may be necessary in its implementation to avoid contamination and limit the transmission of organisms.
- Emphasis on hand hygiene and the use of affordable sterile disposable milk containers that is more convenient are some measures to counter the often reported improper and un-hygienic handling of EBM.
- The paucity of lactational support because of inadequate staffing and limiting its availability to working hours may negatively affect mothers breastfeeding their preterm infants. Improving lactational support services to be more far reaching in coverage to include dedicated nurse counsellors for out-of-office hours and even in extending to the community has been shown to increase breastfeeding success rates in many units.
- Family-centred care with facilities for extended KMC time, longer periods of maternity leave, providing workplace lactation space and support may also increase the success of breastfeeding of the preterm infant.

Chapter 9

Illustrative case series with Q&A

- This chapter presents some of the commonly encountered feeding problems in preterm infants.
- The clinical scenarios presented are real and the management approaches as well as the therapeutic interventions discussed at the end are comprised of the actual action plans and outcomes proposed by the chief author and contributors for each case.
- Questions are posed at different sections of these cases to allow readers to think through each step of the case and suggest the approach that they themselves would take at that stage in management.

Case study 1	Study questions
SD was the smaller twin of a spontaneous monochorionic, diamniotic twin pregnancy. Antenatal scans were normal till 27 weeks when asymmetrical growth retardation developed, with reversal of umbilical Doppler flow. The pregnancy was further complicated with maternal pre-eclampsia and preterm rupture of membranes at 28 weeks. SD was delivered via emergency lower segment caesarean section at 28 weeks for worsening maternal pre-eclampsia. Apgar scores were 3 and 8 at the 1st and 5th minute of life. His birth weight was 1220 g, length 36.5 cm and head circumference was 27.5 cm (10th–50th percentile). He needed NP-CPAP with fraction of inspired oxygen (FiO_2) at 21% for the first 3 days of life.	
Feeding was started on Day 1 of life with minimal enteral feeds (breast milk) and gradually increased. Total parenteral nutrition (TPN) was prescribed for 11 days and he regained birth weight at Day 12 of life. Growth was noted to be faltering by the 3rd week of life despite increasing feeds to 160 ml/kg/day with fully fortified breast milk. As serum sodium was found to be low at 127 mmol/l, oral sodium supplementation was given. No other complications such as chronic lung disease, necrotising enterocolitis (NEC) or sepsis occurred. The infant was discharged at 38 weeks corrected age with a weight of 2.25 kg. Ten weeks later, the weight was 2.75 kg (10th–50th percentile).	1. Would you have started feeds on Day 1? 2. What would have been your approach if the infant still did not achieve optimal growth with fortified breast milk and sodium supplementation? 3. Would you have continued breast milk fortification after discharge? 4. If the mother had no breast milk, what would have been your post-discharge nutrition for this infant?
Case contributed by Dr. Le-Ye Lee and Associate Prof. Jiun Lee, Singapore	

Case study 2

IA was the second twin of a spontaneous dichorionic diamniotic pregnancy. At the 19 weeks foetal scan, IA was noted to be at the < 5th percentile for weight with echogenic bowel detected. The other twin was growing normally with size equivalent to dates throughout the pregnancy. At 25 weeks IA had asymmetrical intrauterine growth retardation (IUGR) and decreased liquor volume was detected. Doppler studies revealed absent end-diastolic flow, with reversal of cerebral perfusion ratio. This persisted throughout the next three scans at 3-weekly intervals. He was delivered via emergency caesarean section at 34 weeks + 5 days. Apgar scores were 7 and 9 at 1 and 5 minutes of life. The birth weight was 861 g; length, 34 cm; and head circumference was 27 cm (all < 3rd percentile). The placenta showed velamentous cord insertion, with no infarction or necrosis. He required NP-CPAP for respiratory support.

During the early post-natal period, the glucose infusion rate (GIR) had to be increased to 9.7 mg/kg/minute to maintain normoglycaemia. Feeds with breast milk were started at 39 hours of life and increased gradually at 10 ml/kg/day. At Day 15, he suffered from *Enterobacter cloacae* septicaemia. Inotropic support and high frequency oscillatory ventilation were needed. Enteral nutrition was stopped when he was acutely ill and parenteral nutrition was restarted. He had 21 days of antibiotic treatment and was discharged only at 44 weeks with a weight of 1884 g (< 3rd percentile). He remained small despite maximising feed volume and supplementation with HMF, nutrient-enriched breast milk substitute and medium-chain triglycerides.

Case contributed by Dr. Le-Ye Lee and Associate Prof. Jiun Lee, Singapore

Study questions

1. Would you have started the feeds earlier?
2. Would you have done the same and stopped feeds when the infant was acutely ill?
3. Would we need to catch up on growth when the infant remains small?

Case study 3

AC was delivered prematurely at 28 weeks. She was delivered via lower segment caesarean section for suspected abruptio placenta with clinical chorioamnionitis. Her birth weight was 1.05 kg. She had mild respiratory distress syndrome and required nasal CPAP. Antibiotics were commenced due to the presence of chorioamnionitis.

On Day 2 of life, she developed abdominal distension. Enteral feeding was not commenced yet at this juncture. There were greenish gastric residuals from her orogastric tube. Her abdominal radiograph showed presence of pneumatosis intestinalis (see figure), and her stool samples were positive for occult blood. The full blood count showed haemoglobin (Hb) 13.4 g/dl, total white cell (TWC) $9.0 \times 10^9/l$, platelets $288 \times 10^9/l$. Her CRP was < 0.07 mg/dl and procalcitonin (PCT) was 0.46 ng/ml.

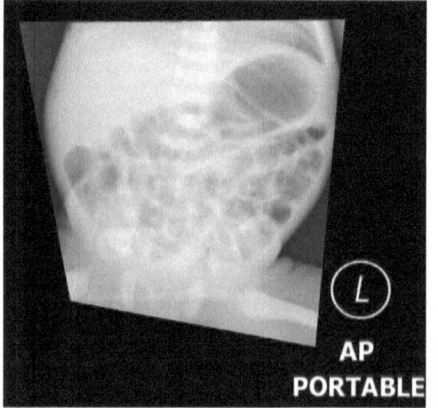

She was kept nil by mouth. TPN was commenced with 0.5 g/kg intralipid, 1 g/kg amino acid and dextrose 10% on the first day. The intralipid was increased to 3 g/kg, amino acid to 4 g/kg and dextrose to 12.5% over 5 days. AC improved clinically. Her abdominal distension and greenish aspirates resolved. Repeated stool samples were negative for occult blood.

Study questions

1. According to Bell's classification, what would this NEC stage be?

2. Would you have started on a different TPN regime?

Case study 3 *(cont'd)*	Study questions
Antibiotics were stopped after one week; her blood culture did not yield any growth. She did not require an increase in respiratory support, and was stable on nasal CPAP with FiO_2 of 21%. She did not receive any other medication apart from antibiotics.	
After one week of being kept nil by mouth, feeding was commenced. She was first given 1 ml/6-hourly pasteurised expressed breast milk (EBM). The feeding frequency was increased to 1 ml/4-hourly, then 1 ml/2-hourly in the subsequent days. After she had tolerated 1 ml/2-hourly feeds, the volume was increased by 1 ml twice a day. AC achieved full oral feeding of 14 ml/2-hourly in about 10 days. Human milk fortifier (HMF) was added to her pasteurised breast milk feeds. She was discharged with the weight of 1.855 kg at Day 52 of life.	3. How long would you have kept this infant nil by mouth? 4. Would you have used pasteurised breast milk? 5. Should HMF be added to breast milk for this infant, and how is HMF associated with NEC?
Case contributed by Dr. Joyce Hong and Prof. Dr. FC Cheah, UKM Medical Centre, Malaysia	

Case study 4

DJ was delivered prematurely at 25 weeks via spontaneous vaginal delivery. Her mother went into spontaneous labour just as the decision to deliver the infant by caesarean section was made, in view of maternal pre-eclampsia and HELLP (haemolysis, elevated liver enzyme levels, and low platelet levels) syndrome. DJ weighed 890 g. She required mechanical ventilation and 2 doses of intratracheal beractant.

At Day 2 of life, she developed abdominal distension. She was still nil by mouth at this stage. Initial abdominal radiograph showed dilated loops of bowel. She was treated with intravenous antibiotics. Her full blood count at that time showed Hb 14.5 g/dl, TWC 6.6 X 10^9/l, platelets 165 X 10^9/l. Her CRP was 0.08 mg/dl and PCT was 0.94 ng/ml. However, DJ's abdominal distension worsened and on Day 6 of life, a repeat abdominal radiograph showed pneumoperitoneum (see figure below). She underwent exploratory laparotomy, where there was a single perforation at mid-jejunum, 20 cm from the duodeno-jejunal junction, with meconium contamination of the peritoneal cavity. She required a jejunostomy.

She was kept nil by mouth and was on TPN. She received 0.5 g/kg intralipid, 1 g/kg amino acid and dextrose 10% on the first day. The intralipid was increased to 3 g/kg, amino acid to 4 g/kg and dextrose to 12.5% over 5 days.

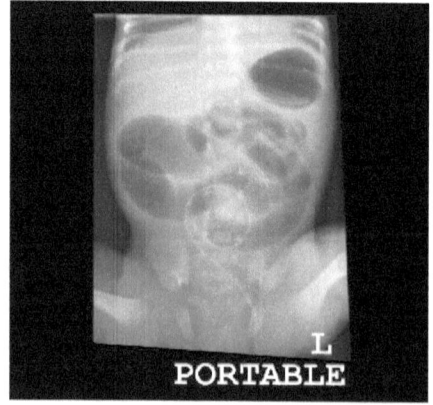

Study questions

Case study 4 (cont'd)

Feeding was commenced about one week after surgery. Initially, she was fed with pasteurised EBM at 1 ml/6-hourly. The frequencies of the feeds were increased from 4-hourly to 2-hourly interval. This was followed by increment in volume of 1 ml each day. However, when she was feeding at about 4 to 5 ml/2-hourly, it was discovered that her stoma losses were increasingly watery and larger in volume than her feeds. She required fluid replacement with Hartmann solution when her stoma losses exceeded 10 ml/kg. She was kept nil by mouth again for a few days till her stoma losses reduced in volume.

When feeding was recommenced, she was given 1 ml/2-hourly of pasteurised breast milk. As she reached a volume of 4 ml/2-hourly, her stoma losses again became more watery and increased in volume. Her feeding was then infused over 1 hour each time, gradually increased to 6 ml/2-hourly. However, that did not help to reduce her stoma losses. A change of feeding was made, whereby she was started on extensively hydrolysed breast milk substitute, but the volume of stoma losses remain unchanged.

Subsequently, she was given a trial of lactose free breast milk substitute. This seemed to help reduce the stoma losses and improve the consistency. Her feeds were still given by infusion over 1 hour. She managed to achieve up to 10 ml/2-hourly feeds. The infusion time was reduced gradually to 45 minutes, 30 minutes, then 15 minutes over the course of about 10 days. She was then successfully given bolus feeds, using lactose-free breast milk substitute. She passed loose stools through her stoma, in normal amounts. At Day 84 of life, she successfully underwent reversal of her jejunostomy. Throughout this period, parenteral nutrition support was still administered in addition to enteral feeding.

At Day 105 of life, when she was getting feeds of 120 ml/kg/day of lactose-free breast milk substitute, DJ was switched back to pasteurised EBM. She was able to tolerate her feeds and there was no change in her stool pattern. At Day 107 of life, she was taken off parenteral nutrition entirely.

DJ was discharged at Day 120 of life, with a weight of 1.8 kg.

Case contributed by Dr. Joyce Soo-Synn Hong and Prof. FC Cheah, UKM Medical Centre, Malaysia

Study questions

1. What was the cause of her increased stoma losses, and how would you have approached this situation?

2. Would you have also used infusion feeds?

3. When would you have transitioned the infant back to breast milk?

Case study 5

RH was a female neonate with birth weight of 690 g (< 10th centile) and was delivered at 26 weeks' gestation. Antenatal scans showed restricted foetal growth with absent end diastolic flow through the umbilical artery. Mother had pregnancy induced hypertension and received two doses of betamethasone 24 hours before delivery. At birth, RH required intubation and ventilatory support for poor respiratory effort. The Apgar scores were 4 and 8 at 1 and 5 minutes respectively. Respiratory distress was managed with surfactant administration, mechanical ventilation followed by extubation to CPAP on Day 3 of life. Antibiotics were ceased at 48 hours as the blood culture results did not indicate sepsis.

A routine surveillance echocardiogram on Day 2 showed a patent ductus arteriosus of 1.8 mm diameter with significant steal in aortic flow. A course of 5 doses of intravenous indomethacin was administered. Follow up echocardiogram on Day 6 confirmed closure of the ductus arteriosus.

Parenteral nutrition was started within 24 hours after birth. Minimal enteral feeds with maternal EBM (10 ml/kg/day) were started on Day 4. Recurrent large bile stained gastric residuals, and abdominal distension with visible 'ropy' bowel loops resulted in frequent stoppage of feeds. Full enteral feed of 150 ml/kg/day was achieved at the post-natal age of 28 days.

On the 35th day of life, RH was noted to have increased gastric aspirates, abdominal distension, with pneumatosis intestinalis on abdominal X-ray. She was treated for NEC. The feeds were stopped, and intravenous vancomycin, gentamycin, and metronidazole were commenced. Progressive metabolic acidosis and worsening of abdominal distension, and fall in platelet counts occurred over the next 24 hours. The repeat X-ray on Day 38 showed free intraperitoneal gas indicative of intestinal perforation (see figure on page 95). The worsening clinical condition and X-ray findings necessitated an exploratory laparotomy. Extensive bowel necrosis

Study questions

1. Would you have started feeds when the infant was on indomethacin? What are your thoughts on indomethacin predisposing the infant to NEC?

2. Would you have started TPN within 24 hours?

3. When would you have started minimal enteral feeds (MEF)?

4. Why should MEF be started as early as Day 1?

5. How would you manage gastric residuals?

Case study 5 (cont'd)

was detected resulting in resection of the terminal sigmoid colon and formation of an ileostomy. Post-operative course was complicated by worsening ventilatory and oxygen requirements, hypotension and metabolic acidosis. Antibiotics were stopped after 8 days. Following gradual recovery, the enteral feeds were reintroduced on Day 48 and full feeds were reached on Day 24 after bowel resection. At the corrected age of 36 weeks, RH was still growth restricted (1746 g, weight < 10th centile).

Abdominal X-ray showing free intraperitoneal gas following intestinal perforation due to NEC.

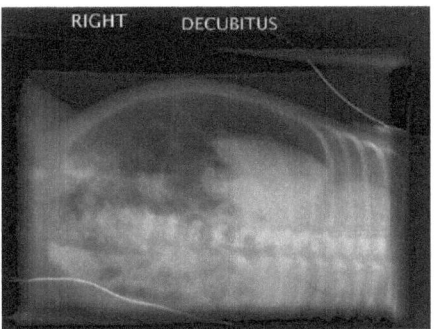

Case contributed by Dr. Girish Deshpande and Prof. Sanjay Patole, Australia

Study questions

6. What are your thoughts on probiotics in preventing NEC?

Case study 6

FSH was a male neonate with birth weight 970 g and was delivered at 26 weeks gestation. The pregnancy was complicated by cervical incompetence, and preterm delivery. Following the spontaneous onset of labour, he required a caesarean in view of breech presentation. Only one dose of steroids was given just before the delivery. At birth, no significant resuscitation was required. Apgar scores were 8 at 1 minute and 9 at 5 minutes respectively.

FSH was initially managed with CPAP but he needed mechanical ventilation from 16 hours until Day 4 of life, and subsequently extubated to CPAP. Two doses of surfactant were given. He received antibiotics for 5 days due to raised infection markers (CRP 22 mg/L and PCT 144.7 μg/L); blood and cerebrospinal fluid (CSF) cultures remained sterile. A routine surveillance echocardiogram on Day 2 showed a patent ductus arteriosus of 1 mm diameter which did not require treatment.

Parenteral nutrition was started within 24 hours after birth. Minimal enteral feeds with maternal EBM (10 ml/kg/day) were started on Day 6. This delay was due to non-availability of breast milk. Lactation consultant support was provided and the mother was commenced on metoclopramide to assist lactation. Feeds were increased by 20 ml/kg/day in the first 2 days and later by 30 ml/kg/day. Breast milk was transitioned to breast milk substitute on Day 8 after discussing with the mother due to non-availability of breast milk. The neonate reached full feeds on Day 12.

On Day 12 of life, he was noted to have abdominal distension, frank blood stained stool, and an episode of blood stained vomiting. Abdominal X-ray showed extensive pneumatosis intestinalis, portal gas shadow and thickened bowel wall confirming NEC Stage II (see figure on page 97). There was no evidence of free air in the peritoneum. He had elevated inflammatory markers thrombocytopenia (104 X 10^9/L) and acidosis. The feeds were stopped, and intravenous vancomycin, gentamycin, and metronidazole were commenced.

Study questions

1. Would you have started MEF earlier even when breast milk was unavailable?

2. Would you have started the mother on a galactagogue such as metoclopramide at this stage?

3. What is your understanding of breast milk substitute and NEC? In this situation, would you have counselled the mother about the use of donor human milk instead?

4. Will you use probiotics to prevent NEC when the neonate is not receiving enteral feeds?

Case study 6 (cont'd)

He also required mechanical ventilation. Although the NEC was initially managed medically, he was transferred to a surgical centre after 4 days, due to persistent low platelet count, raised infection markers and abdominal ultrasound showing localised collection with a non-vascular mass below the liver. A total of 10 cm of necrotic bowel was resected and a colostomy was performed. He tolerated the surgical procedure quite well and post-operative recovery was uneventful.

Abdominal X-ray showing extensive pneumatosis intestinalis and portal gas in NEC

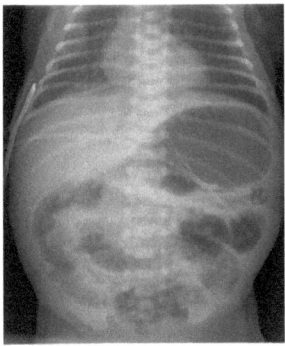

Case contributed by Dr. Girish Deshpande and Prof. Sanjay Patole, Australia

Study questions

Case study 7	Study questions
SH was a female infant, born prematurely at 28 weeks via emergency lower segment caesarean section for breech presentation in labour. The pregnancy was uncomplicated. She was symmetrically small for her gestational age and her physical maturity corresponded to about 30 weeks of gestation. Her birth weight was 1.455 kg, length was 37 cm and head circumference was 28 cm. At birth, she was born "limp" with bradycardia, and required positive pressure ventilation followed by intubation. She was given intratracheal surfactant at 30 minutes of life and connected to mechanical ventilation. The chest radiography showed changes suggestive of respiratory distress syndrome (RDS). She was ventilated for 2 days followed by nasal CPAP for 17 days and high flow nasal cannula for 7 days. She had a patent ductus arteriosus which closed with one course of ibuprofen.	
She was started on TPN via a peripheral inserted central catheter (PICC) from Day 1 of life. Trophic feeding was introduced at Day 3 of life with breast milk substitute (P22) at 2 ml 6 hourly, then at daily increment of 20 ml/kg/day to 30 ml/kg/day. EBM was introduced from Day 5 onwards. She had frequent large amounts of gastric residuals at Day 8 of life which resolved after 6 hours of bowel rest. Enteral feeding was restarted with slower increment of 15 to 20 ml per kg per day and it was tolerated well.	1. In the event that we are unable to start early trophic feeding because breast milk is unavailable, what would your approach be? 2. Would you stop feeds in the presence of large gastric residuals?
Mother's breast milk was analysed using infrared spectrometry. The average breast milk sample profile was as follows: fat 3.6 g/100 ml, crude protein 1.3 g/100 ml, carbohydrate 6.6 g/100 ml, true protein 0.8 g/100 ml, and total calories 63 kcal/100 ml. Breast milk was fortified with HMF at Day 17 of life when SH's enteral feeding reached 140 ml/kg/day. Despite adding HMF into EBM for a week with total fluid intake of 150 ml/kg/day, her weight gain remained poor. Whey protein concentrate (Myotein®) was added at Day 25 of life at 1 to 1.5 g/day, increasing total protein intake to 3.45 g/kg/day from 2.78 g/kg/day. With this, her weight gain improved, and reaching 1.88 kg at Day 46 of life. She was	3. What would you have done when the infant did not grow adequately despite on full enteral feeds (150 ml/kg/day) with EBM? Would you have only considered HMF with no additional protein at this stage?

Case study 7 (cont'd)

discharged well with breastfeeding. On clinic follow-up post-discharge growth rate was satisfactory.

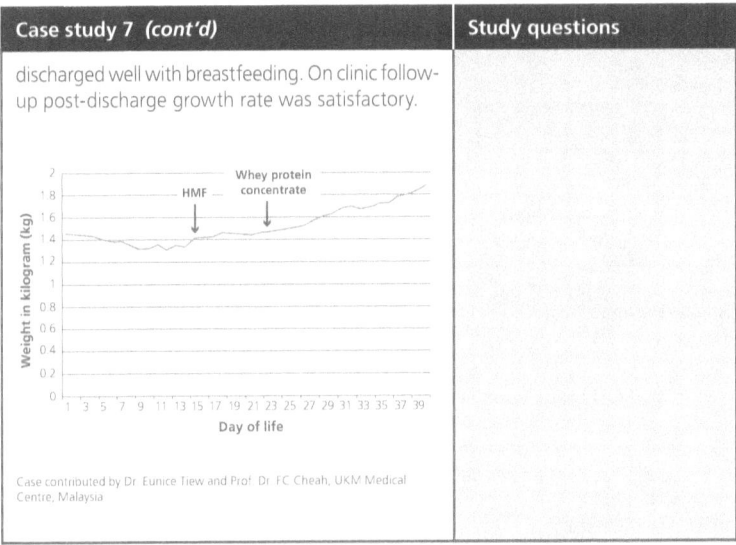

Case contributed by Dr. Eunice Tiew and Prof. Dr. FC Cheah, UKM Medical Centre, Malaysia

Study questions

Case study 8

EC was a female infant, was born at 28 weeks 6 days via emergency caesarean section for unprovoked foetal bradycardia with birth weight of 825 g. Her mother was a 33-year old with essential hypertension and this pregnancy was complicated by pre-eclampsia. Uterine artery Doppler ultrasonography revealed no abnormality in the uteroplacental circulation. A course of antenatal steroid was given at 27 weeks of gestation in anticipation of early delivery. At birth, EC was resuscitated with endotracheal intubation for severe RDS. She was ventilated for 9 days and developed right lung collapse post-extubation. She needed oxygen supplementation with FiO_2 of 25% and was on non-invasive ventilation till Day 55 of life. Her patent ductus arteriosus closed after a course of ibuprofen.

EC was started on TPN via a PICC from Day 1 of life. The starting of enteral feeding was delayed until Day 4 due to persistently high gastric residuals which were brownish, and the unavailability of colostrum. Trophic feeding with EBM was started at 1 ml 6 hourly. However, her abdomen became distended one day after trophic feeding and persistent brownish gastric residuals resumed. She was kept nil by mouth for presumed NEC. There was no temperature instability, metabolic acidosis or occult blood in stools and abdominal radiograph did not show features of NEC. She had a short course of antibiotics for 5 days and feeding was resumed at Day 10 of life. Subsequently, she tolerated her feeding well with slow increment and achieved feeding of 150 ml/kg/day at Day 18 of life. Mother's breast milk was fortified with HMF at Day 19 and additional supplements such as folic acid and multivitamins were started. EC's weight gain in the ward was poor, despite on full feeds with HMF.

Study questions

1. Would you have started feeds earlier despite the brownish gastric residuals?

2. Would you have continued feeds even with persistent brownish residuals?

3. What would the feeding volume advancement rate be if feeds were resumed after a presumptive diagnosis of NEC?

4. What would you do if the infant's weight was still not quite satisfactory despite full feeds at 150 ml/kg/day?

Case study 8 (cont'd)

Mother's breast milk was analysed using infrared spectrometry. On average, her breast milk content profile was as follows: fat 3.2 g/100 ml, crude protein 1.2 g/100 ml, carbohydrate 7.0 g/100 ml, true protein 0.8 g/100 ml, and total calories 62 kcal/100 ml.

Whey protein concentrate was added to the mother's breast milk with targeted protein of 4.5 g/kg/day. EC tolerated the additional protein well with no complications. Her growth rate improved.

At Day 70 of life (approximately 39 weeks corrected age), EC was discharged with a weight of 2.2 kg without needing oxygen supplementation.

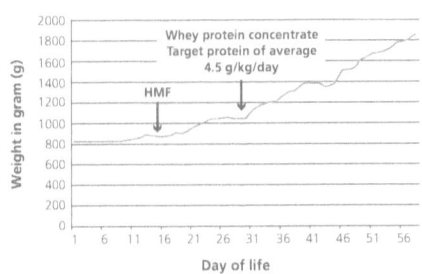

Case contributed by Dr. Eunice Wah-Tin Tiew and Prof. FC Cheah, UKM Medical Centre, Malaysia

Study questions

5. Would you consider periodic bedside breast milk analysis in the NICU? What is your interpretation of this breast milk analysis?

6. What are your thoughts on the protein target of 4.5 g/kg/day on the growth and development of this infant?

Case study 9

CLH was born at 33 weeks via emergency caesarean section for foetal distress. Her mother was a 31-year-old lady with no significant medical history. Her regular antenatal follow-up visits showed a foetus with progressive IUGR and a reduction in amniotic fluid index. Doppler ultrasonography showed a high Uterine Artery Resistive Index (UARI) of 0.72. A course of antenatal steroid was given at 30 weeks of gestation in anticipation of early delivery.

CLH was delivered following premature pre-labour rupture of membranes for 3 days. At birth, she was vigorous with good Apgar scores. She was symmetrically small for gestational age (SGA) with all growth parameters at < 10th percentile for her gestation. Her birth weight was 1100 g, head circumference was 26.5 cm and length was 37 cm.

CLH did not require any respiratory support post-delivery and was nursed in an incubator without oxygen supplementation. Intravenous antibiotics, i.e. crystalline penicillin and gentamicin were commenced in view of prematurity with risk of sepsis. It was stopped after 48 hours as the laboratory markers were not suggestive of infection and blood cultures did not grow any organism.

She was initially kept nil by mouth and commenced on Dextrose 10% infusion intravenously. Feeding was started at 20 hours of life via an orogastric tube with breast milk substitute (P22) at 1 ml 2 hourly (MEF of 10 ml/kg/day) while TPN was administered via a PICC. She tolerated her first four feeds but on the fifth feed, she developed high gastric residuals of 3 ml but without abdominal distension. Feeds were resumed after omitting the two subsequent feeds and these were tolerated well. The increment rate in feeding was 20 ml/kg/day at Day 3 and Day 4 of life. From Day 5 onwards, the increment increased to 30 ml/kg/day till a total fluid intake of 150 ml/kg/day was achieved at Day 7, and 180 ml/kg/day at Day 10 of life. Meanwhile, CLH received breast milk feeds supplemented with breast milk substitute. Later,

Study questions

1. Would you have kept a SGA infant without an abnormal umbilical Doppler ultrasonography nil by mouth for a few days after birth?

2. Would you have stopped feeds when there were large volumes of gastric residuals without abdominal distension?

3. How fast would you have advanced the feeding?

Case study 9 (cont'd)

when more mother's own breast milk was available, CLH was exclusively fed with breast milk fortified with HMF from Day 19 of life onwards. There was no high gastric residuals or abdominal distension or evidence of NEC from this point.

CLH made good progress, tolerated all her feeds and was gaining weight satisfactorily. Feeding via orogastric tube was continued till Day 29 of life (corrected age of 37 weeks), after which breastfeeding was introduced. At Day 32 of life, she was discharged home to her parents at the weight of 1.8 kg (see figure below), exclusive breastfed.

CLH's growth chart:

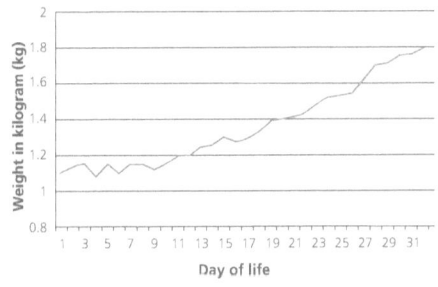

Case contributed by Dr. Eunice Tiew and Prof. Dr. FC Cheah, UKM Medical Centre, Malaysia

Study questions

4. Would you consider post-discharge supplementation of breastfeeding by fortifying EBM or adding a post-discharge formula (PDF)?

Case study 10

LJY was delivered at 34 weeks of gestation via emergency lower caesarean section for IUGR and her birth weight was 1.34 kg. She was one of the triplets conceived successfully by in-vitro fertilisation. The other two were monochorionic diamniotic twins. Serial ultrasound showed growth discrepancy between the twins from 25 weeks of gestation onward, thus antenatal steroids were given at 26 and 33 weeks of gestation in anticipation of early delivery.

LJY was delivered with good Apgar scores and did not require any respiratory support at birth. In view of the history of IUGR, feeding was started gradually with a mixture of breast milk substitute, 24 kcal/oz formula (P24) and EBM. On Day 6 of life, she had recurrent asymptomatic hypoglycaemia requiring multiple intravenous boluses of Dextrose 10% with increments in GIR up to 9 mg/kg/min. Her total fluid intake was increased up to 200 ml/kg/day per oral. Complex glucose polymers (Carborie®) 4.5 g/day was added to her feeds to maintain her blood glucose within the normal range. Despite this, her blood glucose levels were low intermittently. IV hydrocortisone 3.5 mg/kg BD was started on Day 17 of life. Following this, her blood glucose normalised and IV hydrocortisone was ceased after tapering it over 1 week. Added Carborie® was gradually withheld. Her insulin, C-peptide, cortisol level and thyroid function were normal. Both serum ammonia and lactate results were also within normal ranges and the absence of metabolic acidosis did not support an underlying inborn error of metabolism.

She was discharged well on Day 28 of life with a weight of 1.925 kg.

Case contributed by Dr. Wan Nurulhuda bt. Wan Md. Zin and Prof. FC Cheah, UKM Medical Centre, Malaysia

Study questions

1. Would you have used a caloric dense breast milk substitute such as a 22 kcal/oz (P22) or 24 kcal/oz (P24) formula when initiating feeds e.g. for MEF?

2. What would be your approach in managing the feeds for an infant who is hypoglycaemic?

3. What would your approach be if the infant still had hypoglycaemia despite optimising the feeding either enterally and/or parenterally?

Suggested answers and treatment plans to case study questions

Please note that the references are in the footnote at the end of each section.

Case study 1

1. **Would you have started feeds on Day 1?**

    Many would not start feeds early for this case because the infant was premature, growth retarded, and there was evidence of reverse umbilical Doppler flow, suggesting a compromised blood flow to the gastrointestinal tract (GIT). However, we started feeds from Day 1, using breast milk for better tolerance.

    The fear of starting feeds early is due to the perceived risk of NEC but there is evidence to show that there was no added risk with early feeds especially with breast milk[1] (see chapter on enteral feeding - Chapter 2), as seen in this case. Nevertheless, as the infant is considered high risk (less than 29 weeks at birth), feeds should be advanced slowly (15–20 ml/kg/day).

    Breast milk fed to these infants also need to be fortified. But in addition to fortification, this particular infant required sodium chloride supplementation. This could be due to an increased demand for sodium with rapid growth.

2. **What would have been your approach if the infant still did not achieve optimal growth with fortified breast milk and sodium supplementation?**

    Some would push the total fluids higher to 180 ml/kg/day but this could result in large volumes that may jeopardise the feed tolerance from abdominal over distension and also respiratory embarrassment. Many of these infants also may have ongoing or resolving lung disease that may not adjust well to the increased fluid intake.

    An alternative suggestion is to assess the amount of protein intake by analysing the milk or measuring blood urea level. If growth is suboptimal, whey protein can be added into the milk feeds to concentrate the feeds by increasing the protein and monitoring blood urea level to ensure it is not > 5 mmol/L.

3. **Would you have continued breast milk fortification after discharge?**

    For these infants, as the mothers would have been asked to room-in for exclusive breastfeeding before the infant is discharged, we can evaluate whether the infant is able to latch and suck on the breast. Some would discharge the infant with just exclusive breastfeeding, but this may cause growth to falter and poor bone mineralisation, affecting the infant's linear growth, especially among the at risk groups of infants. Therefore, fortification post-discharge may be necessary. Advise the mother to express milk several times a day for the HMF to be added. If we opt not to fortify, monitor the growth of the infant carefully and check the calcium and phosphorus balance as an indicator of bone mineralisation status. The risk of growth failure and insufficient bone mineralisation, and therefore poor linear growth is more likely in at risk infants of < 1500 g and < 32 weeks gestation.

4. **If the mother had no breast milk, what would have been your post-discharge nutrition for this infant?**

   We can use a PDF as it has higher protein and mineral contents than the usual term breast milk substitute. A term breast milk substitute should not be used for a preterm infant discharged from the nursery. There is no real evidence to show that a PDF is superior in terms of neurocognitive benefits but it has been suggested to be better for linear growth[2] (see chapter on post-discharge feeding - Chapter 6).

---

1. Morgan J, Bombell S, McGuire W. Early trophic feeding versus enteral fasting for very preterm or very low birth weight infants. *Cochrane Database Syst Rev.* 2013;3:CD000504. doi:10.1002/14651858.CD000504.pub4; **2.** Fewtrell MS, Prentice A, Jones SC, Bishop NJ, Stirling D, Buffenstein R, et al. Bone mineralization and turnover in preterm infants at 8-12 years of age: the effect of early diet. *J Bone Miner Res.* 1999;14:810-20.

Case contributed by Dr. Le-Ye Lee and Associate Prof. Jiun Lee, Singapore

Case study 2

1. **Would you have started the feeds earlier?**

   The attending neonatologist for this particular case delayed feeding because the infant was at high risk for NEC. However, there is increasing evidence to promote initiating feeds for such infants within the first 24 hours without added risk.

2. **Would you have done the same and stopped feeds when the infant was acutely ill?**

   There is no evidence to show that if an infant is septic, he/she cannot be fed, although there is a tendency for the infant to have feeding intolerance in such situations. Adjust the volume and advance feeds based on the infant's tolerance. Parenteral nutrition is vital to complement the reduced enteral feeding that the infant is subjected to because of his illness.

   Neonatologists also tend to omit lipids from TPN, but this is not beneficial for the infant. When acutely ill, infants need essential fatty acids for cell membrane synthesis with an increase in cell turnover, as well as prostaglandins that are involved in immune-modulation during the inflammation cascade of a sepsis episode. Include lipids but at reduced rates as tolerance is lower when infants are acutely ill. Adjust lipids by measuring triglyceride (TG) levels only during the acutely ill period, as neonatologists are starting to move away from the regular measurement of TG levels for TPN, a historical practice which has not been backed-up with sufficient evidence (see chapter on parenteral nutrition - Chapter 1).

3. **Would we need to catch up on growth when the infant remains small?**

   Some infants remain small at a particular percentile, and they should be followed up as such to ensure that they do not cross the percentile too rapidly during their first year. These are infants who may remain small because of intrauterine programming. Therefore, if an infant remains small even after feeds are maximised, they should be allowed to remain small. If growth is too rapid, the infant could develop metabolic syndrome later in life. Nevertheless, as this SGA infant is also preterm, we should use all avenues to help him achieve better growth and offer him the opportunity to increase growth to more than the 3rd percentile. This is because better growth in a preterm infant may be associated with positive neurocognitive outcomes, with many receptive of this as an importantly advantageous benefit when balanced against the risk of developing metabolic syndrome later in life.

Case contributed by Dr. Le-Ye Lee and Associate Prof. Jiun Lee, Singapore

Case study 3

1. **According to Bell's classification, what would this NEC stage be?**

   Stage IIB (moderately ill)

2. **Would you have started on a different TPN regime?**

   For the preterm infant, we should start amino acid at 3 g/kg instead of 1 g/kg. We can start at high levels even when the infant is acutely ill to overcome increased catabolism in such situations. In fact, amino acid of 1.5 g/kg is minimum to overcome a negative energy balance and prevent catabolism occurring in the sick premature infant.

3. **How long would you have kept this infant nil by mouth?**

   Currently, there is no evidence to indicate how long an infant with NEC should be kept nil by mouth. In the author's practice, infants with NEC Stage I are kept nil by mouth for a maximum of 5 days. If there is presence of pneumatosis as in this case, the infant is kept nil by mouth for 7–10 days, with repeat abdominal X-ray at the end of the nil by mouth period to rule out the extension or deterioration of NEC before resuming feeds. Keeping nil by mouth and administering TPN are crucial in the management of an infant with NEC. Also antibiotics that are active against anaerobes, and intermittent decompression of the bowel with an orogastric tube should be provided. In summary, the strategy is to "rest" the bowel by keeping the infant nil by mouth, provide antibiotic cover and decompress the bowel by free flow with intermittent aspiration through an orogastric tube, and wait for the bowel to heal before resuming feeds.

   In very ill cases and infants with apnoeic episodes, I would electively ventilate them rather than continue with CPAP as theoretically CPAP may aggravate the bowel distension and increase transmural pressure in the bowel wall risking progression to perforation.

4. **Would you have used pasteurised breast milk?**

   Breast milk (including pasteurised donor breast milk) has been shown to be superior to breast milk substitutes in protecting the infant from NEC.[1] In this case, pasteurised milk from the infant's mother was used. Some suggest that the infant gut should be protected from potentially high levels of pathogenic bacteria that could be present in some mother's milk in the absence of close and regular surveillance. As this infant was recovering from NEC, the attending neonatologist did not want to increase the risk of the infant being colonised by pathogenic bacteria (see chapter on cultural practices - Chapter 8; as well as the studies on the contamination of breast milk.[2,3])

   There is relative preservation of the major nutrients in breast milk with pasteurisation (see chapter on breastfeeding - Chapter 3). However, live cells, antibodies, and probiotics (see chapter on probiotics - Chapter 7) that could be beneficial in protecting the premature gut practically disappear with pasteurisation.

5. **Should HMF be added to breast milk for this infant, and how is HMF associated with NEC?**

HMF is added when the infant is fed at least 50% of his total feeds (70–80 ml/kg) enterally. In the author's setting, HMF is added at 75% (120 ml/kg). We should be mindful that HMF can also increase the osmolarity of feeds, leading to feeding intolerance in some infants. Therefore tailor HMF supplementation to the individual needs of the infants based on their tolerance. Always abide by the manufacturer's instructions in using the appropriate amounts of HMF to EBM ratio.

As cow-milk based HMF has been reported to reduce the protective effects of breast milk, the use of human-based HMF is suggested. But human HMF is not widely available and only one study has shown it to be better than cow-milk based HMF.[4] There is no evidence of increased NEC with HMF.[5]

1. Herrmann K, Carroll K. An exclusively human milk diet reduces necrotizing enterocolitis. *Breastfeed Med.* 2014;9(4):184-902; **2.** Boo NY, Nordiah AJ, Alfizah H, Nor-Rohaini AH, Lim VK. Contamination of breast milk obtained by manual expression and breast pumps in mothers of very low birth weight infants. *J Hosp Infect.* 2001;49(4):274-81; **3.** Dahaban NM, Romli MF, Roslan NR, Kong SS, Cheah FC. Bacteria in expressed breast milk from mothers of premature infants and maternal hygienic status. *Breastfeed Med.* 2013;8(4):422-3; **4.** Sullivan S, Schanler RJ, Kim JH, Patel AL, Trawoger R, Kiechl-Kohlendorfer U, et al. An exclusively human milk-based diet is associated with a lower rate of necrotizing enterocolitis than a diet of human milk and bovine milk-based products. *J Pediatr.* 2010;156(4):562-7 e1; **5.** Kuschel CA, Harding JE. Multicomponent fortified human milk for promoting growth in preterm infants. *Cochrane Database Syst Rev.* 2004(1):CD000343

Case contributed by Dr. Joyce Hong and Prof. Dr. FC Cheah, UKM Medical Centre, Malaysia

Case study 4

1. **What was the cause of her increased stoma losses, and how would you have approached this situation?**

   Because of short gut syndrome and a reduced absorptive surface area, infants would often have diarrhoea or watery stools when feeds are progressively increased.

   Feeds should be reduced but exercise care as reduced volumes could lead to electrolyte imbalance and dehydration, as well as hypoglycaemia. Adjust supplementation with TPN if enteral feeds are reduced. In some instances, the infant may benefit from loperamide, an agent used to treat diarrhoea. Loperamide will slow down bowel movement, leading to increased transit time of feeds in the gut for absorption and reduced losses. Monitor these losses, as one may need to replace the excessive fluid losses and correct electrolyte imbalances with preferably supplementary parenteral nutrition.

2. **Would you have also used infusion feeds?**

   Infusing feeds gradually may theoretically reduce stoma losses by increasing the transit time, but this is rarely helpful. Extensively hydrolysed breast milk substitute (see Appendix 2) may help in some instances as it is pre-digested, therefore the gut does not need to break it down into smaller particles to be digested, and is less osmogenic. However, this approach did not work in this case.

   This infant had lactose intolerance caused by lactase deficiency. She was able to tolerate lactose free breast milk substitute.

3. **When would you have transitioned the infant back to breast milk?**

   "Challenge" the gut gradually and progressively with breast milk, overlapping with lactose free breast milk substitute. The aim is to get the infant to fully feed on breast milk again. In my practice, I would gradually overlap feeds by introducing 3-5 ml of breast milk incrementally as the "challenge".

   Case contributed by Dr. Joyce Soo-Synn Hong and Prof. FC Cheah, UKM Medical Centre, Malaysia

Case study 5

1. **Would you have started feeds when the infant was on indomethacin? What are your thoughts on indomethacin predisposing the infant to NEC?**

   Some do not start feeds when infants are on indomethacin, but there is no evidence to show that feeds should not be given. Pharmacologically, indomethacin may reduce gut microcirculation and perfusion.

   There have been reports associating indomethacin to a higher risk of NEC,[1] as well as with isolated gastric perforation.[1] These could be the fears that influence many to avoid feeds during indomethacin therapy.

2. **Would you have started TPN within 24 hours?**

   We should start TPN within 24 hours, as IV drip alone is insufficient to provide the energy requirement. There is sufficient evidence this is the preferred method with more benefits than risks (see chapter on parenteral nutrition - Chapter 1).

3. **When would you have started MEF?**

   We should start MEF from Day 1, and preferably with breast milk. But in this case, we should exercise caution and feeds should not exceed 20 ml/kg because of the multiple risk factors such as extreme prematurity, ELBW and abnormal Doppler.

4. **Why should MEF be started as early as Day 1?**

   MEF is important to reduce the risk of sepsis related to parenteral nutrition and to establish full enteral feeding early with a more rapid weight gain (see chapter on enteral feeding - Chapter 2).

5. **How would you manage gastric residuals?**

   Although we should assess gastric residuals, it should not be over-emphasised especially if the infant has no other ominous abdominal signs (see chapter on breastfeeding - Chapter 3).

   For infants with feeding intolerance, consider adding prokinetics (see chapter on feeding IUGR infants - Chapter 5).

6. **What are your thoughts on probiotics in preventing NEC?**

   Probiotics are known to reduce the risk of definite NEC in the preterm (Gestation < 34 weeks) VLBW neonates (see chapter on probiotics - Chapter 7). However, the current data on the effects of probiotics in extremely preterm (gestation < 28 weeks) neonates, especially those who are also growth restricted, is limited. Further research is necessary to assess the safety and efficacy of probiotics in this population of neonates that deserve them the most. Many practitioners resist introducing this therapy because of a "wait-and-see" approach for further development and evidence to emerge in this area specifically on the preferred species of probiotic or their combination, and also the dosing concentration, frequency and duration.

   In my practice, I would also like to improve the uptake in the use of raw breast milk containing natural probiotics first before introducing this as an add-on therapy.

Additional comments: Overall this case represents the difficulties in enteral feeding and the high risk of NEC in extremely preterm neonates. Consequences of NEC including the need for surgery, and survival with short bowel syndrome and extrauterine growth restriction are also highlighted, especially those with IUGR. It also illustrates that definite (Stage II) NEC commonly presents at around 3rd week of life in extremely preterm neonates, and its progression to Stage III (advanced/surgical) usually occurs in 2–3 days after the diagnosis.

1. Irmesi R, Marcialis MA, Anker JV, Fanos V. Non-steroidal anti-inflammatory drugs (NSAIDs) in the management of patent ductus arteriosus (PDA) in preterm infants and variations in attitude in clinical practice: a flight around the world. *Curr Med Chem.* 2014;21(27):3132-52.

Case contributed by Dr. Girish Deshpande and Prof. Sanjay Patole, Australia

Case study 6

1. **Would you have started MEF earlier even when breast milk was unavailable?**

   Yes, the feeding algorithm (see chapter on enteral feeding - Chapter 2) suggests that MEF should be started within 24 hours after birth, even when breast milk is unavailable. In most cases, colostrum in small amounts should already be produced. Use breast milk substitutes or preferably donor breast milk if available. Some prefer to go "slow" and be cautious if there is no breast milk by starting with less hyperosmolar feeds such as diluted breast milk substitute or even hydrolysed formula expecting improved tolerance. There have been anecdotal reports and small studies reporting an advantage.

2. **Would you have started the mother on galactagogue such as metoclopramide at this stage?**

   Evidence shows that lactation improves with galactagogue two weeks after delivery.[1] The recommended galactagogue is domperidone (see chapter on breastfeeding - Chapter 3).

3. **What is your understanding of breast milk substitute and NEC? In this situation, would you have counselled the mother about the use of donor human milk instead?**

   This case highlights the importance of breast milk feeding for the prevention of NEC. Not all neonatal units have access to breast milk bank although very low birth weight (VLBW) neonates fed with breast milk substitute have increased risk of NEC. "One-to-one" sharing of EBM in the NICU as discussed in chapter 3, may be an alternative approach that can be explored further. In this case, one could also argue that feeds were increased quickly than recommended (> 20 ml/kg/day), particularly when supplemental breast milk substitute was required. The current evidence also supports the use of standardised feeding regimens in preterm VLBW neonates to reduce the risk of NEC.

   Other simple and well established strategies include early preferential feeding with breast milk, and antenatal steroids for prevention of NEC in preterm neonates. A full course of steroids is associated with less NEC in the preterm infant. In this high risk preterm infant who was less than 1 kg at birth, did not receive full course of steroids, had a patent ductus arteriosus, and did not receive breast milk, as well as had his feeds advanced too rapidly, probiotics may be offered to reduce the risk of NEC.

4. **Will you use probiotics to prevent NEC when the neonate is not receiving enteral feeds?**

   Probiotics can be considered provided that the neonate is not unwell and there are no bile aspirates.

---

1. Donovan TJ, Buchanan K. Medications for increasing milk supply in mothers expressing breast milk for their preterm hospitalised infants. *Cochrane Database Syst Rev.* 2012;3:CD005544.

Case contributed by Dr. Girish Deshpande and Prof. Sanjay Patole, Australia.

Case study 7

1. **In the event that we are unable to start early trophic feeding because breast milk is unavailable, what would your approach be?**

    Many mothers delivering prematurely will not be able to produce sufficient breast milk in the initial few days after birth, and therefore donor milk or breast milk substitutes may be necessary.

    We can use donor breast milk if available, or breast milk substitutes such as hydrolysed protein breast milk substitutes which may be better tolerated.[1]

2. **Would you stop feeds in the presence of large gastric residuals?**

    Gastric residuals are usually benign (see chapter on enteral feeding - Chapter 2). Often times neonatologists have unfounded fears and choose to err on the "safe" side thus, may be omitting feeds too quickly. Preferably stop feeds only when other abdominal symptoms/signs are also present. If there are no other symptoms/signs, modify the feeding regime, "watch-and-see" and then resume feeds as tolerated.

3. **What would you have done when the infant did not grow appropriately despite on full enteral feeds (150 ml/kg/day) with EBM? Would you have only considered HMF with no additional protein at this stage?**

    We propose doing a breast milk analysis. If the analysis reveals insufficient calories in the milk, modify the feeds accordingly. If a milk analysis is unavailable, adjust fortification by adding HMF with protein up to 4–4.5 g/kg/day (as per ESPGHAN recommendation on protein intake for preterm infants), and use blood urea as a guide (≤ 5 mmol/l is the cut-off point). Many would increase the volume of the feeds from 150 ml/kg/day to 180 ml/kg/day and even 200 ml/kg/day instead of fortifying the feeds. However, increasing the volume for preterm infants may run the risk of fluid retention for some infants that may impair lung function, especially in infants with underlying heart or lung disease. If the infant has bronchopulmonary dysplasia (BPD), or a recently closed patent ductus arteriosus (PDA), we may not want to increase the fluid volume too much. In such instances, a preferred alternative may be to concentrate the feeds by adding HMF and whey protein concentrate.

---

[1]. Mihatsch WA, Franz AR, Hogel J, Pohlandt F. Hydrolyzed protein accelerates feeding advancement in very low birth weight infants. *Pediatrics.* 2002;110(6):1199-203.

Case contributed by Dr. Eunice Tiew and Prof. Dr. FC Cheah, UKM Medical Centre, Malaysia

Case study 8

1. **Would you have started feeds earlier despite the brownish gastric residuals?**

    Yes, after determining the cause of the brownish gastric residuals and ruling out any pathological condition. In many cases this may be altered swallowed blood in amniotic fluid. Do an APT test to confirm (refer for method in footnote on page 29) With feeding, the altered blood should clear with no further signs of deterioration (see chapter on enteral feeding - Chapter 2). If there is no breast milk, donor breast milk or lower osmolarity/hydrolysed breast milk substitutes could be used.

2. **Would you have continued feeds even with persistent brownish residuals?**

    In many instances, feeds are stopped because of the fear of NEC. However, in the author's experience, as NEC related mortality is high, NEC is often presumed until proven otherwise in most instances even with vague abdominal signs and will be treated as such. The bowel is "rested" for 5 days before feeds are resumed. TPN is mandatory for nutritional support during this period.

3. **What would the feed advancement rate be if feeds are resumed after a presumptive diagnosis of NEC?**

    Based on the multiple risk factors of extreme prematurity, ELBW and prior NEC, we would recommend advancement not exceeding 20 ml/kg/day.

4. **What would you do if the infant's weight was still not quite satisfactory despite full feeds at 150 ml/kg/day?**

    Increasing the volume further in this case, may be less appropriate as it potentially reopens the patent ductus arteriosus and also may impair lung function, as an infant who needs oxygen supplementation and respiratory support is sensitive to perturbation in lung function secondary to pulmonary congestion. Breast milk analysis may shed some light on the infant's suboptimal growth attributable to low calories in the milk consumed.

5. **Would you consider periodic bedside breast milk analysis in the NICU? What is your interpretation of this breast milk analysis?**

    Mother's milk can vary in energy content even on a day to day basis and at different post-conceptional ages (see chapter on breastfeeding - Chapter 3). Bedside analysis of mother's milk is a useful tool and in this case, it showed that the mother's milk was relatively low in calories and protein content. If HMF is not able to achieve the recommended protein intake, the use of whey protein may be additionally supplied to achieve the target of 4.0 to 4.5 g/kg/day as recommended by European Society of Paediatric Gastroenterology, Hepatology and Nutrition (ESPGHAN).

6. **What are your thoughts on the targeted protein of 4.5 g/kg/day on the growth and development of this infant?**

   Some are concerned that whey protein concentrate may increase the feed's osmolarity, leading to feeding intolerance. However, emerging evidence showed improved growth especially in infants less than 30 weeks and less than 1 kg at birth.[1,2] Various whey protein concentrate prepared for this purpose are available in the market (see Appendix 2). HMF added into breast milk will on average supply added protein of up to 3.5 g/kg/day. A further 0.5-1 g/kg/day protein, preferably in whey form, may be necessary for the extremely preterm and ELBW infants based on current recommendation.

1. Moya F, Sisk PM, Walsh KR, Berseth CL. A new liquid human milk fortifier and linear growth in preterm infants. *Pediatrics*. 2012;130(4):e928-35. **2.** Cheah FC. A randomized controlled trial comparing the effects of individualizing and standardized fortification of expressed breast milk on the growth of preterm infants in the NICU. Poster presented at the 12th World Congress Perinatal Medicine: 3–6 November 2015, Madrid, Spain.

Case contributed by Dr. Eunice Wah-Tin Tiew and Prof. FC Cheah, UKM Medical Centre, Malaysia

Case study 9

1. **Would you have kept a SGA infant without an abnormal umbilical Doppler ultrasonography nil by mouth for a few days after birth?**

   Preferably feeds should still be started early.[1] There is no evidence to indicate that withholding feeds will reduce the risk of NEC in this at risk group. Refer to the feeding protocol the author has used for this group of infants in a study which showed early feeding was not associated with a significant increased risk in feeding intolerance or NEC than delayed feeding for > 48 hours (see chapter on enteral feeding - Chapter 2). This protocol was developed to incorporate a more gradual advancement rate in feed increment.

2. **Would you have stopped feeds when there were large volumes of gastric residuals without abdominal distension?**

   Feeds are recommended not to be ceased entirely, but to be modified accordingly based on tolerance. (see chapter on enteral feeding - Chapter 2, and case study 7).

3. **How fast would you have advanced the feeding?**

   Based on the author's unit protocol (see chapter on enteral feeding - Chapter 2 and chapter on strategies and challenges in feeding the preterm infant with intrauterine growth retardation - Chapter 5) and the protocol used in the Abnormal Doppler Enteral Prescription Trial (ADEPT) trial[1,2] (see Chapter 5), initial advancement is recommended not to be > 20 ml/kg.

   Additional comment: With the early introduction and "pushing" on with feeds despite the high gastric residuals, this infant was able to successfully achieve full feeding relatively early (by Day 10 of life), and her weight increased at a satisfactory rate (mean of 23 g of weight gained per day), despite the SGA status.

4. **Would you consider post-discharge supplementation of breastfeeding by fortifying EBM or using a PDF?**

   As this infant was SGA, < 34 weeks and VLBW, I would recommend 2-3 feeds per day of EBM with added HMF (refer chapter on post-discharge nutrition - Chapter 6) or in the event that the mother has a lack of breast milk, supplement some feeds using PDF. This approach hopefully could allow for some catch-up growth that should be carefully monitored. It is hoped that with improved growth, better neurocognitive gains for this infant can also be achieved.

1. Bakon FA, Cheah FC, Ishak S, Wan Puteh SE. Premature small for gestational age infants: early versus delayed feeding. Poster presented at 19th Annual PSM Perinatal Congress 2012; **2.** Leaf A, Dorling J, Kempley S, McCormick K, Mannix P, Linsell L, et al. Early or delayed enteral feeding for preterm growth-restricted infants: a randomized trial. Pediatrics. 2012;129:e1260-8.

Case contributed by Dr. Eunice Tiew and Prof. Dr. FC Cheah, UKM Medical Centre, Malaysia

Case study 10

1. **Would you have used a caloric dense breast milk substitute such as a 22 kcal/oz (P22) or 24 kcal/oz (P24) formula when initiating feeds e.g. for MEF?**

   Preferably use colostrum/EBM, but if unavailable, the initial use of P22 formula may be better tolerated because of its slightly lower osmolarity. Many practitioners just use standard (term) breast milk substitute because of the initial small volumes for MEF primarily to prime the gut.

2. **What would be your approach in managing the feeds for an infant who is hypoglycaemic?**

   As SGA infants have poor glycogen stores, they can readily develop hypoglycaemia (plasma glucose concentration of 1.7–2.8 mmol/l)[1] [see chapter on feeding IUGR infants - Chapter 5]. The first step, if the infant can suck, is to offer a high caloric feed given enterally. Increase the volume of feeds as appropriate and the extras may need to be gavage fed. Because breast milk has lower calories, we may have to use a caloric dense breast milk substitute (P24) and increase the volume of intake enterally to 180 ml/kg/day, even 200 ml/kg/day. The limiting factor is when the infant vomits and cannot tolerate this larger volume of feeds.

   Often times doctors tend to start IV very quickly forgetting that there is a healthy functioning gut. Only if the above fails to achieve normoglycaemia, one may have to initiate parenteral fluids with glucose of 10%–12.5% through peripheral intravenous cannula. For glucose of 15%, a central line for access in the form of an umbilical vein catheter or PICC is required. As the caloric content of mother's breast milk frequently varies, it is sometimes challenging to use it as feeds to rectify the low sugar levels in an infant with hypoglycaemia. If glucose control is not too difficult to rectify, the first options for feeds should still be mother's own milk, and add on calories with HMF, whey protein or a glucose polymer complex (e.g. Carborie®) as required before resorting to caloric dense breast milk substitutes or parenteral fluids.

3. **What would your approach be if the infant still had hypoglycaemia despite optimising the feeding either enterally and parenterally?**

   Utilise pharmacotherapy, such as hydrocortisone or somatostatin to increase glucose levels. Glucagon is not preferred for infants with growth retardation as they lack glycogen stores for mobilisation to energy sources.

   Additional comments: In this case, the glucose polymer was added into the feeds gradually as the resulting increase in osmolarity may lead to feeding intolerance. Despite this the infant still did not receive sufficient glucose, leading to persistent hypoglycaemia that was corrected with pharmacotherapy. A proactive feeding regimen in moderately preterm SGA infants has been shown to significantly reduce the risk of hypoglycaemia.[2] The GIR is useful to monitor the glucose needs during the acute period of hypoglycaemia and to predict the recovery phase when the GIR starts to decrease and fall back to the normal range of 6-8 mg/kg/min.

1. Wight N, Marinelli KA. ABM clinical protocol #1: guidelines for blood glucose monitoring and treatment of hypoglycemia in term and late-preterm neonates, revised 2014. *Breastfeed Med.* 2014;9(4):173-9; **2.** Zecca E, Costa S, Barone G, Giordano L, Zecca C, Maggio L. Proactive enteral nutrition in moderately preterm small for gestational age infants: a randomized clinical trial. *J Pediatr.* 2014;165(6):1135-9 e1.

Case contributed by Dr. Wan Nurulhuda bt. Wan Md. Zin and Prof. FC Cheah, UKM Medical Centre, Malaysia

Appendices

Appendix 1: Sample of TPN order form from UKM Medical Centre

UNIVERSITI KEBANGSAAN MALAYSIA MEDICAL CENTRE
PHARMACY DEPARTMENT ASEPTIC SERVICES (03-9145 6702/6701)
TPN ORDER FORM FOR *PRE-TERM NEONATES*

Name		R/N		Ward		Bed no.	
				Sex	M		F
Weight	Date of birth		Age	Route	Central		Peripheral

Diagnosis

FIGURES ARE PER *KG* PER 24 HOURS

DATE :						NOTES :
REGIMEN ORDERED						
(1) Total daily fluid (ml)						
(2) Total other B fluid (ml)						
(1)-(2) Fluid for TPN (ml)						
DOCTOR'S NAME						
SIGNATURE						
Pager Number						

STANDARD REGIMEN / 24hrs[1]	1	2	3	4	5	6
Protein (g/kg)	3.0	3.0	3.5	3.5	4.0	4.0
Carbohydrate (%)	7.5%	10%	10%	12.5%	12.5%	15%
Peditrace™ (ml/kg)	1	1	1	1	1	1
Sodium (mmol/kg)[2]	1	1	1	3	3	3
Potassium (mmol/kg)	2.5	2.5	2.5	2.5	2.5	2.5
Calcium (mmol/kg)	0.6	0.6	0.6	0.6	0.6	0.6
Magnesium (mmol/kg)	0.3	0.3	0.3	0.3	0.3	0.3
Phosphate (mmol/kg)	0.15	0.4	0.4	0.4	0.4	0.4
Solivite™ (ml/kg)	1	1	1	1	1	1
Vitalipid™ N Infant (ml/kg)	1	1	1	1	1	1
Lipid (g/kg)	1.0	1.5	2.0	2.5	3.0	3.5

[1]: Regimen 1 for day 1 on TPN, regimen 2 for day 2 and so forth, regimen 6 for day 6 onwards.
[2]: For neonates < 1kg birth weight, a starting amount of 1mmol/kg for sodium is recommended. Otherwise, sodium content can be altered as required.

Additional notes:
- Dextrose (10–12.5 %) recommended for peripheral line
- For term babies (less than 2 months old) **protein content exceeding 3gm/kg/day is not recommended**
- Regimens will be supplied as 2-in-1 bags with separate lipid syringes, to be infused together

Appendix 1 *(cont'd)*

DATE: ALTERATION in REGIMEN						
Protein *(g/kg)*						
Carbohydrate *(%)*						
Peditrace™ *(ml/kg)*						
Sodium *(mmol/kg)*[2]						
Potassium *(mmol/kg)*						
Calcium *(mmol/kg)*						
Magnesium *(mmol/kg)*						
Phosphate *(mmol/kg)*						
Solivite™ *(ml/kg)*						
Vitalipid™ N Infant *(ml/kg)*						
Lipid *(g/kg)*						

REF: Journal of Pediatric Gastroenterology & Nutrition 41: S12-S18 Nov 2005 ESPGHAN GUIDELINES
Last edited: 1.10.2012

Accuracy and monitoring to be verified against pharmacy and manufacturer's information.

Appendix 2: Tables comparing compositions of breast milk, breast milk additives and breast milk substitutes (milk formula)

Selected nutrient composition of breast milk by gestation

Nutrients per 100 ml

Breast milk	Energy (kcal)	Protein (g)	Fat (g)	Docosahexaenoic acid weight percentage of total FA)	Lactose (kcal)	Oligosaccharides (g)	Calcium (mg)	Phosphate (mg)
Day 1-3								
Term	54	2.0	1.8	1.08	5.6	1.6	26	11
Preterm	49	2.7	2.2	1.09	5.1	-	25	10
Day 4-7								
Term	66	1.6	2.6	0.68	6.0	1.9	26	13
Preterm	71	1.7	3.0	0.93	6.3	2.1	27	13
Week 2								
Term	66	1.3	3.0	NA	6.2	1.9	28	15
Preterm	71	1.5	3.5	NA	5.7	2.1	25	15
Week 3-4								
Term	66	1.1	3.4	0.52	6.7	1.6	27	16
Preterm	77	1.4	3.5	0.65	6.0	1.7	25	14
Week 5-6								
Term	63	1.0	3.6	NA	6.1	1.4	25	16
Preterm	70	1.1	3.2	NA	5.8	-	28	13
Week 7-9								
Term	63	0.9	3.4	NA	6.5	1.3	26	16
Preterm	76	1.1	3.3	NA	6.3	-	30	14
Week 10-12								
Term	63	1.0	3.4	NA	6.7	-	27	16
Preterm	-	1.0	3.7	NA	6.8	-	29	12

NA: information unavailable

Source: Gidrewicz DA, Fenton TR. A systematic review and meta-analysis of the nutrient content of preterm and term breast milk. BMC Pediatr. 2014;14:216; Aydin I, Turan Ö, Aydin FN, Koç E, Hirfanoğlu IM, Akyol M, et al. Comparing the fatty acid levels of preterm and term breast milk in Turkish women. Turk J Med Sci. 2014;44(2):305-10.

Selected nutrition composition of breast milk by stages

Nutrients per 100 ml

Breast milk	Energy (kcal)	Protein (g)	Fat (g)	Lactose (kcal)	Calcium (mg)	Phosphate (mg)
Colostrum						
Term	54	2.0	1.8	5.6	26	11.0
Preterm	49	2.7	2.2	5.1	25	9.5
Mature milk						
Term	63	1.0	3.4	6.5	26	16.0
Preterm	73	1.1	3.3	6.2	29	12.8

Source: Gidrewicz DA, Fenton TR. A systematic review and meta-analysis of the nutrient content of preterm and term breast milk. BMC Pediatr. 2014;14:216.

Appendix 2 *(cont'd)*

Acid amino composition of breast milk

Nutrients (mg/100 ml)

Acid amino	Gestation period	
	Term	Preterm
Histidine	34.5	41.7
Leucine	159.3	192.4
Lysine	107.8	134.7
Phenylalanine	63.8	79.1
Valine	83.3	117.1
Tryptophan	21.4	32.1
Threonine	68.4	102.1
Methionine	21.1	27.8
Isoleucine	84.0	95.5
Arginine*	64.9	93.8
Alanine	56.8	90.9
Aspartate	130.1	174.4
Tyrosine*	68.8	88.3
Proline	128.2	153.0
Glycine*	41.7	55.0
Serine	90.2	111.8
Glutamate	252.9	305.3
Cysteine*	28.0	32.0

*essential amino acids for preterm infants

Source: Zhang Z, Adelman AS, Rai D, Boettcher J, Lönnerdal B. Amino acid profiles in term and preterm human milk through lactation: a systematic review. Nutrients. 2013;5(12):4800-21.

Appendix 2 *(cont'd)*

Selected nutrient composition of preterm breast milk substitutes available in Malaysia

Nutrients per 100 ml

Breast milk substitutes	Energy (kcal)	Protein (g)	Fat (g)	Carbohydrate (g)	Oligosaccharides (g)	Docosahexaenoic acid (mg)	Calcium (mg)	Phosphate (mg)
Dumex Mamex Premature®	80	2.6	3.9	8.5	0.76	15.2	100	56
Enfamil® Premature	80	2.4	4.1	8.8	NA	13.7	96	54
Enfalac A+ Post Discharge®	75	2.0	3.9	7.7	NA	12.7	82	48
Nestle PreNAN®	80	2.0	4.1	9.0	NA	15.7	122	71
Similac Neosure®	74	1.9	4.1	7.7	NA	6.0	78	46
S-26 LBW GOLD®	82	2.2	4.4	8.4	NA	17	101	61

NA: information not available

Selected nutrient composition of human milk fortifiers

Nutrients per 100 ml

Human milk fortifiers	Energy (kcal)	Protein (g)	Fat (g)	Carbohydrate (g)	Oligosaccharides (g)	Docosahexaenoic acid (mg)	Calcium (mg)	Phosphate (mg)
Enfamil® Human Milk Fortifier	14	1.1	1.0	< 0.40	NA	NA	90	50
SIMILAC® Human Milk Fortifier	14	1.0	0.36	1.8	NA	NA	117	67
S-26 SMA HMF®	15	1.0	0.16	2.32	NA	NA	92	44

NA: information not available

Appendix 3: Growth charts

UK-WHO growth chart for boys (0-2 years)

Boys: 23-42 weeks of gestation

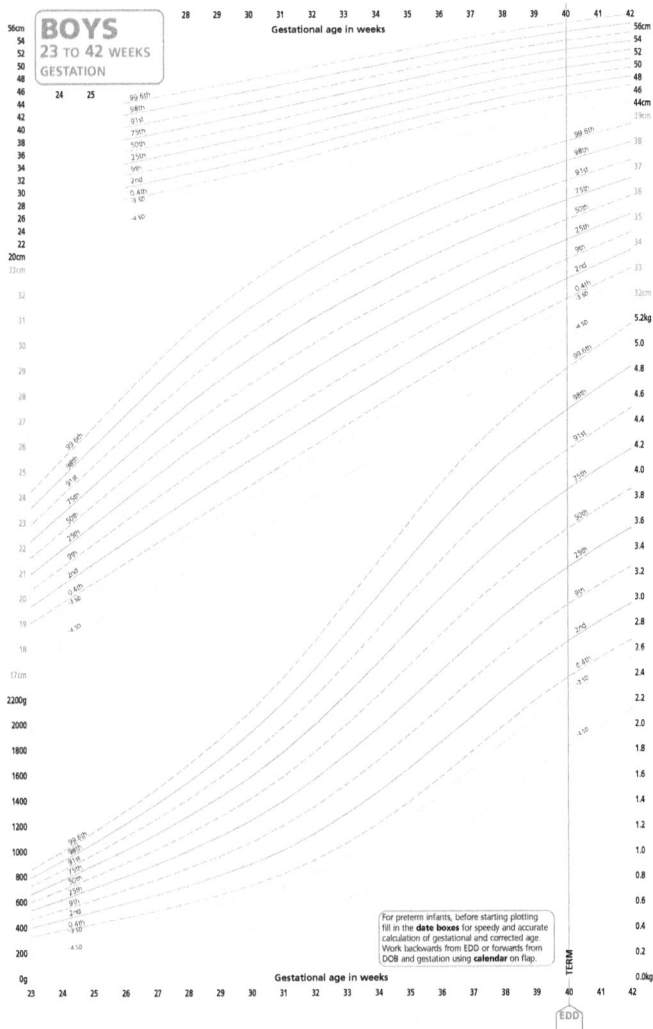

Reprinted from http://www.rcpch.ac.uk/system/files/protected/page/A4%20Boys%200-4YRS%20(4th%20Jan%202013).pdf , Boys UK-WHO chart (0-2 years), Accessed October 2015, with permission from Royal College of Paediatrics and Child Health.

Appendix 3 *(cont'd)*

UK-WHO growth chart for boys (0-2 years)

Boys: 2 weeks to 6 months

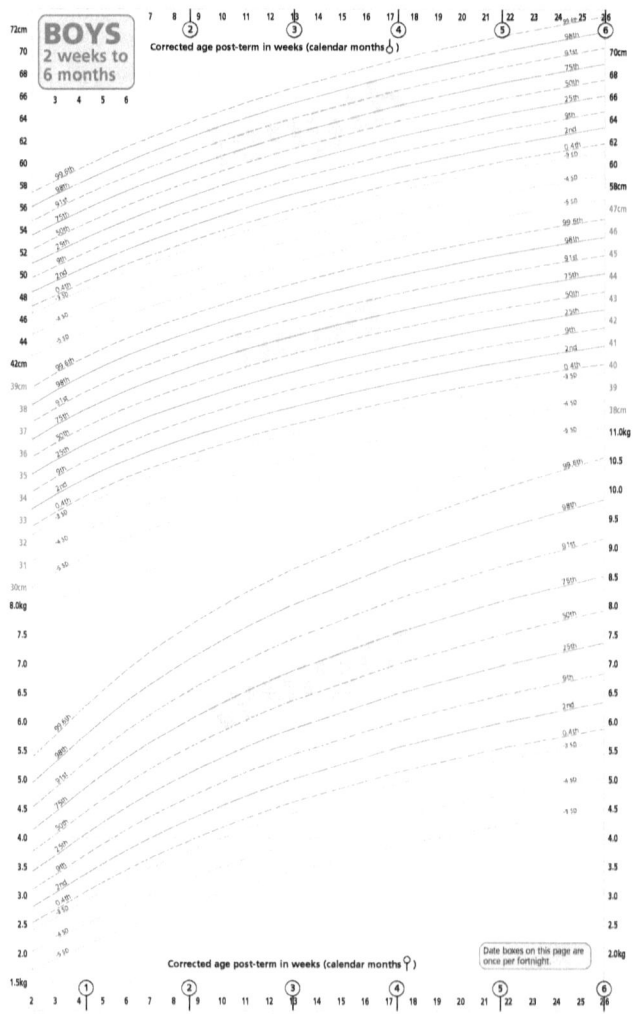

Reprinted from http://www.rcpch.ac.uk/system/files/protected/page/A4%20Boys%200-4YRS%20(4th%20Jan%202013).pdf , Boys UK-WHO chart (0-2 years), Accessed October 2015, with permission from Royal College of Paediatrics and Child Health.

Appendix 3 *(cont'd)*

UK-WHO growth chart for boys (0-2 years)

Boys: 6 months to 2 years

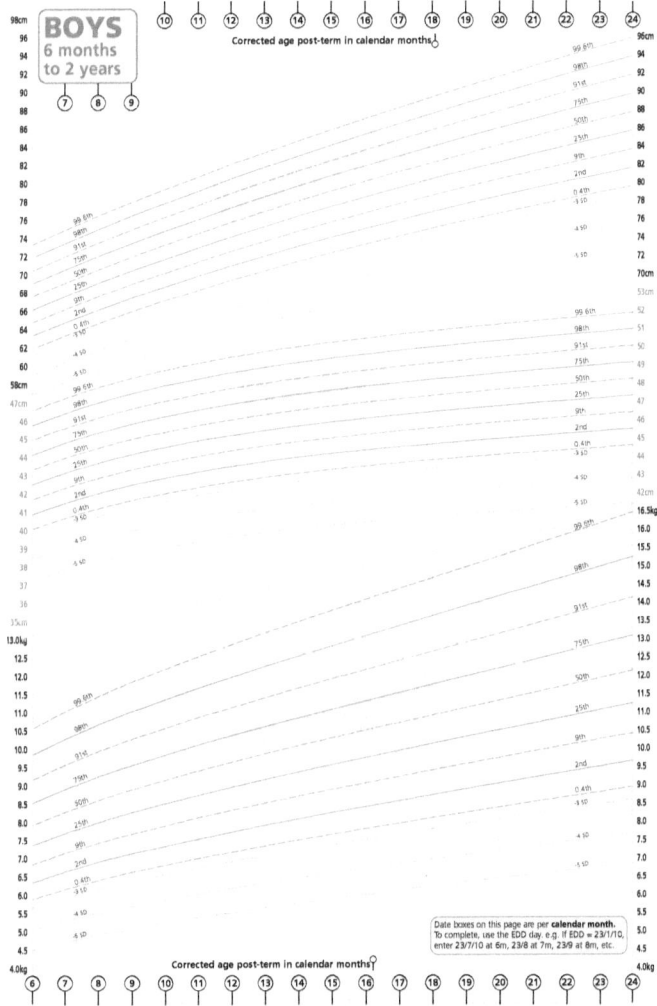

Reprinted from http://www.rcpch.ac.uk/system/files/protected/page/A4%20Boys%200-4YRS%20(4th%20Jan%202013).pdf , Boys UK-WHO chart (0-2 years), Accessed October 2015, with permission from Royal College of Paediatrics and Child Health.

Appendix 3 *(cont'd)*

UK-WHO growth chart for girls (0-2 years)

Girls: 23 to 42 weeks of gestation

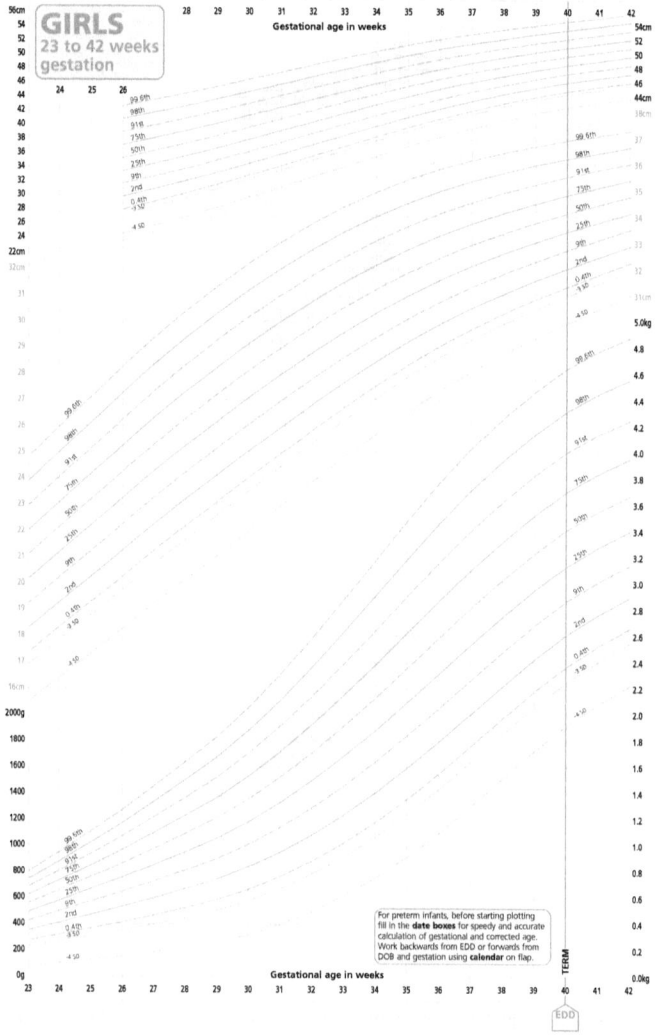

Appendix 3 *(cont'd)*

UK-WHO growth chart for girls (0-2 years)

Girls: 2 weeks to 6 months

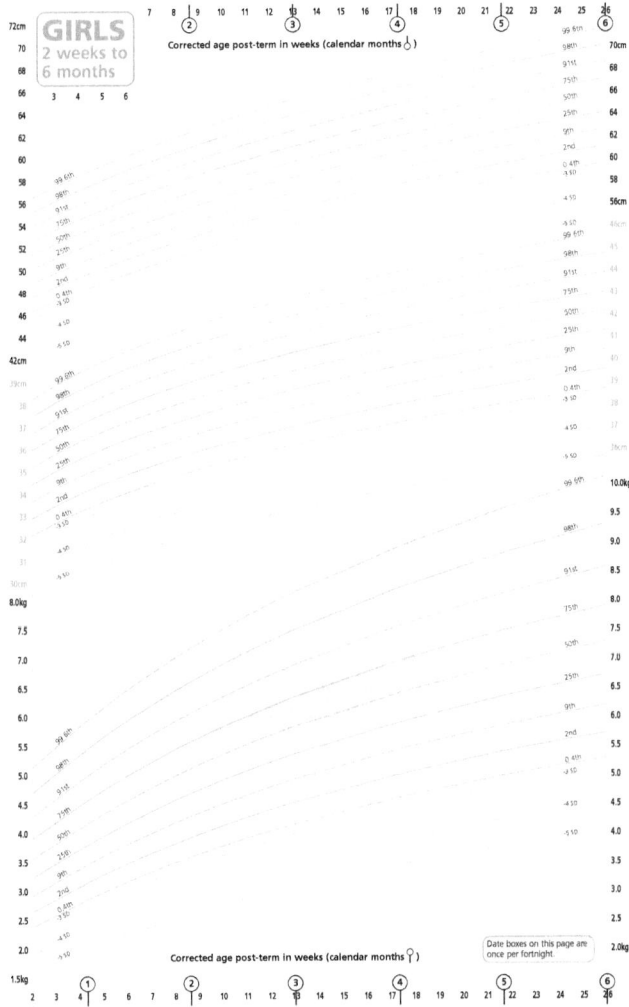

Appendix 131

Appendix 3 *(cont'd)*

UK-WHO growth chart for girls (0-2 years)

Girls: 6 months to 2 years

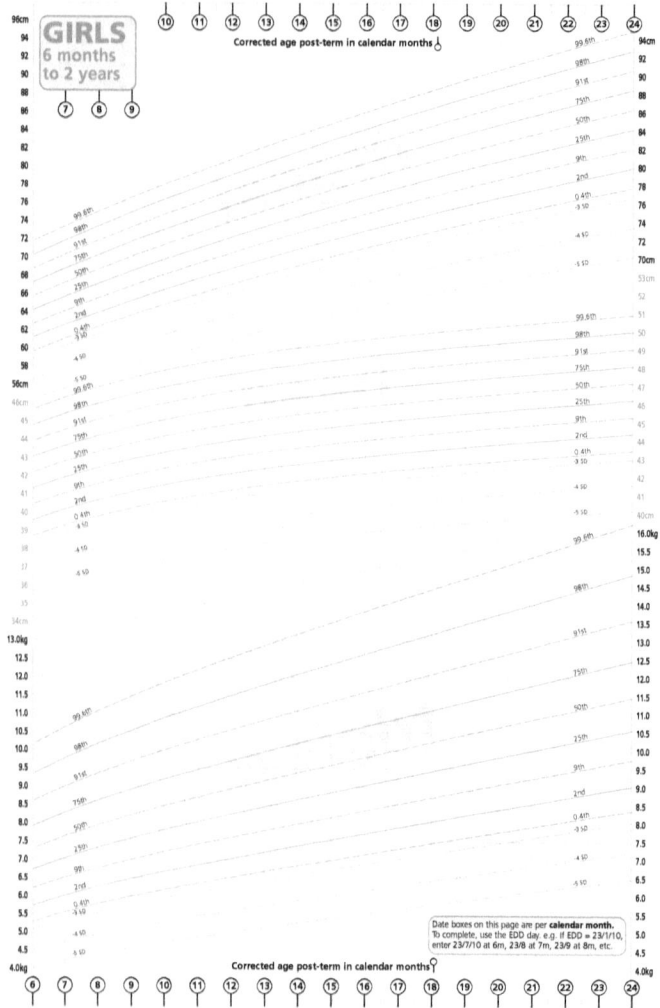

Appendix 3 (cont'd)

2013 Foetal-infant growth chart for preterm infants

Boys

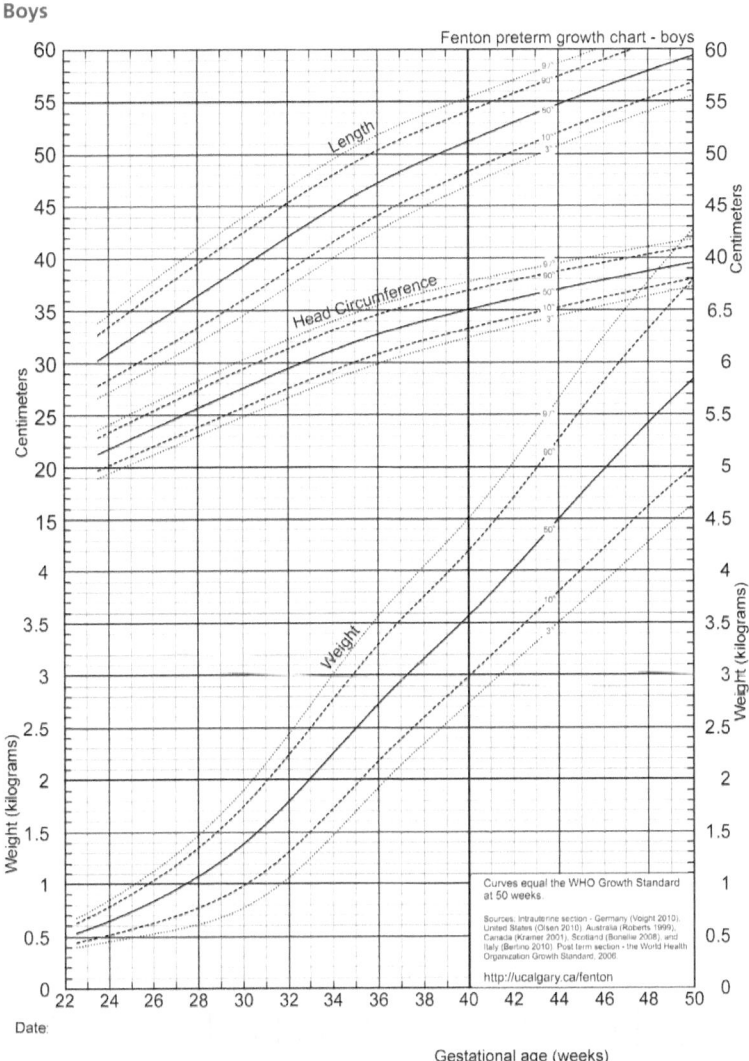

Appendix 3 *(cont'd)*

2013 Foetal-infant growth chart for preterm infants

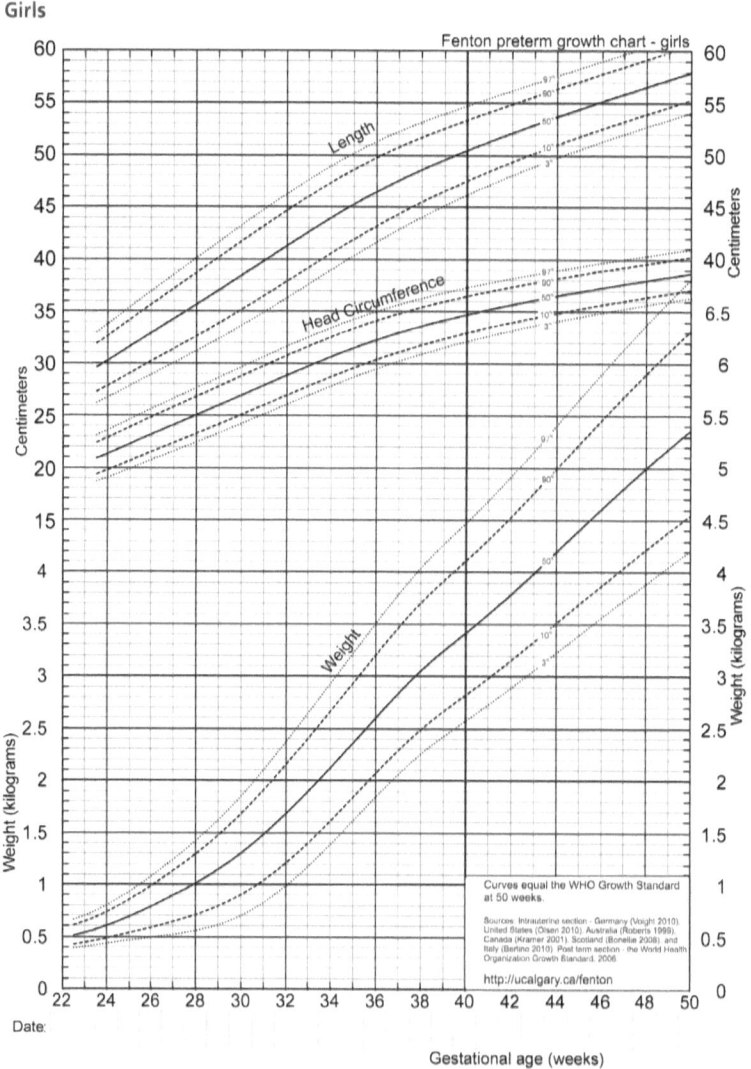

Reprinted from BMC Pediatrics, Vol 13(59), Fenton TR, *et al.*, A systematic review and meta analysis to revise the Fenton growth chart for preterm infants, 2013, with permission from BioMed Central.

References

1. Indrio F, Riezzo G, Cavallo L, Di Mauro A, Francavilla R. Physiological basis of food intolerance in VLBW. *J Matern Fetal Neonatal Med.* 2011;24 Suppl 1:64-6.
2. Neu J. Gastrointestinal development and meeting the nutritional needs of premature infants. *Am J Clin Nutr.* 2007;85:629S-34S.
3. Commare CE, Tappenden KA. Development of the infant intestine: implications for nutrition support. *Nutr Clin Pract.* 2007;22:159-73.
4. Dusick AM, Poindexter BB, Ehrenkranz RA, Lemons JA. Growth failure in the preterm infant: can we catch up? *Semin Perinatol.* 2003;27:302-10.
5. Ziegler EE, Thureen PJ, Carlson SJ. Aggressive nutrition of the very low birthweight infant. *Clin Perinatol.* 2002;29:225-44.
6. Agostoni C, Buonocore G, Carnielli VP, De Curtis M, Darmaun D, Decsi T, et al. Enteral nutrient supply for preterm infants: commentary from the European Society of Paediatric Gastroenterology, Hepatology and Nutrition Committee on Nutrition. *J Pediatr Gastroenterol Nutr.* 2010;50(1):85-91.
7. Thureen PJ, Hay WW. Early aggressive nutrition in preterm infants. *Semin Neonatol.* 2001;6:403-15.
8. Gross SJ, Eckerman CO. Normative early head growth in very-low-birth-weight infants. *J Pediatr.* 1983;103:946-9.
9. Hack M, Breslau N, Fanaroff AA. Differential effects of intrauterine and postnatal brain growth failure in infants of very low birth weight. *Am J Dis Child.* 1989;143:63-8.
10. Moyses HE, Johnson MJ, Leaf AA, Cornelius VR. Early parenteral nutrition and growth outcomes in preterm infants: a systematic review and meta-analysis. *Am J Clin Nutr.*2013;97:816-26.
11. Morisaki N, Belfort MB, McCormick MC, Mori R, Noma H, Kusuda S, et al. Brief parenteral nutrition accelerates weight gain, head growth even in healthy VLBWs. *PLoS One.* 2014;9:e88392.
12. Hussain Imam HMS, Ng HP, Thomas T. Paediatric Protocols for Malaysian Hospitals (3rd ed.). Ministry of Health Malaysia. Available at http://www.mpaweb.org.my/file_dir/6549703650eae1487f6fb.pdf (Accessed November 2015). .
13. ESPGHAN. Guidelines on PN:Complications. *J Pediatr Gastr Nutr.* 2005;41:S76-S84
14. Simmer K, Rakshasbhuvankar A, Deshpande G. Standardised parenteral nutrition. *Nutrients.* 2013;5:1058-70.
15. Shulman RJ, Phillips S. Parenteral nutrition in infants and children. *J Pediatr Gastroenterol Nutr.* 2003;36:587-607.
16. National Health Service UK. Parenteral nutrition. Available at https://www.networks.nhs.uk/nhs-networks/staffordshire-shropshire-and-black-country-newborn/documents/Parenteral%20nutrition%202009-11.pdf. (Accessed October 2015).
17. Velaphi S. Nutritional requirements and parenteral nutrition in preterm infants. *Afr J Clin Nutr.* 2011;24(3):S27-31.
18. Poindexter BB, Langer JC, Dusick AM, Ehrenkranz RA. Early provision of parenteral amino acids in extremely low birth weight infants: relation to growth and neurodevelopmental outcome. *J Pediatr.* 2006;148:300-5.

19. Premji S, Fenton T, Sauve R. Does amount of protein in formula matter for low-birthweight infants? A Cochrane systematic review. *JPEN J Parenter Enteral Nutr.* 2006;30:507-14.
20. Stephens BE, Walden RV, Gargus RA, Tucker R, McKinley L, Mance M, et al. First-week protein and energy intakes are associated with 18-month developmental outcomes in extremely low birth weight infants. *Pediatrics.* 2009;123:1337-43.
21. Zlotkin SH, Bryan MH, Anderson GH. Intravenous nitrogen and energy intakes required to duplicate in utero nitrogen accretion in prematurely born human infants. *J Pediatr.* 1981;99:115-20.
22. Premji SS, Fenton T, Sauve RS. Higher versus lower protein intake in formula-fed low birth weight infants. *Cochrane Database of Systematic Reviews.* 2006;1. Art No: CD003959.
23. Van Goudoever JB, Colen T, Wattimena JL, Huijmans JG, Carnielli VP, Sauer PJ. Immediate commencement of amino acid supplementation in preterm infants: effect on serum amino acid concentrations and protein kinetics on the first day of life. *J Pediatr.* 1995;127:458-65.
24. de Boo HA, Harding JE. Protein metabolism in preterm infants with particular reference to intrauterine growth restriction. *Arch Dis Child Fetal Neonatal Ed.* 2007;92:F315-F319
25. ESPGHAN. Guidelines on PN: Energy. *J Pediatr Gastr Nutr.* 2005;41:S76-S84.
26. Rivera A, Bell EF, Bier DM. Effect of intravenous amino acids on protein metabolism of preterm infants during the first three days of life. *Pediatr Res.* 1993;33:106-11.
27. Hay WW, Jr. Aggressive Nutrition of the Preterm Infant. *Curr Pediatr Rep.* 2013;1(4).
28. Uthaya S, Liu X, Babalis D, et al. Nutritional Evaluation and Optimisation in Neonates (NEON) trials of amino acid regimen and intravenous lipid composition in preterm parenteral nutrition: a randomised double-blind controlled trial. *Efficacy Mech Eval.* 2016;3(2).
29. ESPGHAN. Guidelines on PN: Lipids. *J Pediatr Gastr Nutr.* 2005;41:S19-S27.
30. González-Contreras J, Villalobos Gámez JL, Gómez-Sánchez AI, García-Almeida JM, Enguix Armanda A, Rius Díaz F, et al. Cholestasis induced by total parenteral nutrition: effects of the addition of Taurine (Tauramin®) on hepatic function parameters; possible synergistic action of structured lipids (SMOFlipid®). *Nutr Hosp.*2012;27(6):1900-7.
31. Korver AM, Walther FJ, van der Molen AJ, de Beaufort AJ. Serious complications of umbilical venous catheterisation. *Ned Tijdschr Geneeskd.* 2007;151(40):2219-23.
32. Grizelj R, Vukovic J, Bojanic K, Loncarevic D, Stern-Padovan R, Filipovic-Grcic B, et al. Severe liver injury while using umbilical venous catheter: case series and literature review. *Am J Perinatol.* 2014;31(11):965-74.
33. Bakon FA, Cheah FC. Shareena I, Sharifa EWP. Premature small for gestational age infants: early versus delayed feeding. Poster presented at 19th Annual PSM Perinatal Congress 2012.
34. Morgan J, Bombell S, McGuire W. Early trophic feeding versus enteral fasting for very preterm or very low birth weight infants. *Cochrane Database Syst Rev.* 2013;3:CD000504.
35. Konnikova Y, Zaman MM, Makda M, D'Onofrio D, Freedman SD, Martin CR. Late Enteral Feedings Are Associated with Intestinal Inflammation and Adverse Neonatal Outcomes. *PLoS One.* 2015;10(7):e0132924.
36. Klingenberg C, Embleton ND, Jacobs SE, O'Connell LAF, Kuschel CA. Enteral feeding practices in very preterm infants: an international survey. *Arch Dis Child Fetal Neonatal Ed.* 2012;97:F56-61.
37. Leaf A, Dorling J, Kempley S, McCormick K, Mannix P, Linsell L, et al. Early or delayed enteral feeding for preterm growth-restricted infants: a randomized trial. *Pediatrics.* 2012;129:e1260-8.
38. Siddell EP, Froman RD. A national survey of neonatal intensive-care units: criteria used to determine readiness for oral feedings. *J Obstet Gynecol Neonatal Nurs.*1994;23:783-9.
39. Leaf A, Dorling J, Kempley S, McCormick K, Mannix P, Brocklehurst P. ADEPT - Abnormal Doppler Enteral Prescription Trial. *BMC Pediatr.* 2009;9:63.
40. Morgan J, Young L, McGuire W. Slow advancement of enteral feed volumes to prevent necrotising enterocolitis in very low birth weight infants. *Cochrane Database Syst Rev.* 2013;3:CD001241.

41. National Institute for Health Research, United Kingdom. Speed of increasing milk feeds trials. NCT01727609. Available at: https://clinicaltrials.gov/ct2/show/NCT01727609. Accessed in April 2016.
42. Anderson DM, Kliegman RM. The relationship of neonatal alimentation practices to the occurrence of endemic necrotizing enterocolitis. *Am J Perinatol.* 1991;8:62-7.
43. Dani C, Pratesi S, Barp J. Continuous milk feeding versus intermittent bolus feeding in preterm infants. *Early Hum Dev.* 2013;89 Suppl 2:S11-2.
44. Lucas A, Bloom SR, Aynsley-Green A. Gut hormones and 'minimal enteral feeding'. *Acta Paediatr Scand.* 1986;75:719-23.
45. Aynsley-Green A, Adrian TE, Bloom SR. Feeding and the development of enteroinsular hormone secretion in the preterm infant: effects of continuous gastric infusions of human milk compared with intermittent boluses. *Acta Paediatr Scand.* 1982;71(3):379-83.
46. World Health Organization. Optimal feeding of low-birth-weight infants. 2006. Available at http://apps.who.int/iris/bitstream/10665/43602/1/9789241595094_eng.pdf. (Accessed October 2015).
47. Mihatsch WA, Franz AR, Hogel J, Pohlandt F. Hydrolyzed protein accelerates feeding advancement in very low birth weight infants. *Pediatrics.* 2002;110(6):1199-203.
48. Torrazza RM, Parker LA, Li Y, Talaga E, Shuster J, Neu J. The value of routine evaluation of gastric residuals in very low birth weight infants. *J Perinatol.* 2015;35(1):57-60.
49. Li YF, Lin HC, Torrazza RM, Parker L, Talaga E, Neu J. Gastric residual evaluation in preterm neonates: a useful monitoring technique or a hindrance? *Pediatr Neonatol.* 2014;55(5):335-40.
50. Mihatsch WA, von Schoenaich P, Fahnenstich H, Dehne N, Ebbecke H, Plath C, *et al.* The significance of gastric residuals in the early enteral feeding advancement of extremely low birth weight infants. *Pediatrics.* 2002;109(3):457-9.
51. Mihatsch WA, Franz AR, Lindner W, Pohlandt F. Meconium passage in extremely low birthweight infants and its relation to very early enteral nutrition. *Acta Paediatr.* 2001;90(4):409-11.
52. Poets CF. Gastroesophageal reflux: a critical review of its role in preterm infants. *Pediatrics.* 2004;113:e128-32.
53. van Wijk MP, Benninga MA, Dent J, Lontis R, Goodchild L, McCall LM, *et al.* Effect of body position changes on postprandial gastroesophageal reflux and gastric emptying in the healthy premature neonate. *J Pediatr.* 2007;151:585-90, 90.e1-2.
54. US Food and Drug Administration. Consumer Updates : FDA Expands Caution About SimplyThick. Available at http://www.fda.gov/ForConsumers/ConsumerUpdates/ucm256250.htm. (Accessed October 2015).
55. Kennedy KA, Tyson JE, Chamnanvanikij S. Early versus delayed initiation of progressive enteral feedings for parenterally fed low birth weight or preterm infants. *Cochrane Database Syst Rev.* 2000(2):CD001970.
56. Crook M. Haemoglobin in stools from neonates: measurement by a modified Apt-test. *Med Lab Sci.* 1991;48(4):346-7.
57. Callen J, Pinelli J. A review of the literature examining the benefits and challenges, incidence and duration, and barriers to breastfeeding in preterm infants. *Adv Neonatal Care.* 2005;5:72-88; quiz 9-92.
58. Stelwagen K, van Espen DC, Verkerk GA, McFadden HA, Farr VC. Elevated plasma cortisol reduces permeability of mammary tight junctions in the lactating bovine mammary epithelium. *J Endocrinol.* 1998;159:173-8.
59. Zettl KS, Sjaastad MD, Riskin PM, Parry G, Machen TE, Firestone GL. Glucocorticoid-induced formation of tight junctions in mouse mammary epithelial cells in vitro. *Proc Natl Acad Sci U S A.* 1992;89:9069-73.
60. Hoppu U, Kalliomäki M, Laiho K, Isolauri E. Breast milk--immunomodulatory signals against allergic diseases. *Allergy.* 2001;56 Suppl 6:23-6.

61. Walker A. Breast milk as the gold standard for protective nutrients. *J Pediatr.* 2010;156:S3-7.
62. Tomicić S, Johansson G, Voor T, Björkstén B, Böttcher MF, Jenmalm MC. Breast milk cytokine and IgA composition differ in Estonian and Swedish mothers-relationship to microbial pressure and infant allergy. *Pediatr Res.* 2010;68:330-4.
63. Boyd CA, Quigley MA, Brocklehurst P. Donor breast milk versus infant formula for preterm infants: systematic review and meta-analysis. *Arch Dis Child Fetal Neonatal Ed.* 2007;92(3):F169-75.
64. McGuire W, Anthony MY. Donor human milk versus formula for preventing necrotising enterocolitis in preterm infants: systematic review. *Arch Dis Child Fetal Neonatal Ed.* 2003;88(1):F11-4.
65. Herrmann K, Carroll K. An exclusively human milk diet reduces necrotizing enterocolitis. *Breastfeed Med.* 2014;9(4):184-90.
66. Hoey C, Ware JL. Economic advantages of breast-feeding in an HMO: setting a pilot study. *Am J Manag Care.* 1997;3(6):861-5.
67. Ball TM, Wright AL. Health care costs of formula-feeding in the first year of life. *Pediatrics.* 1999;103(4 Pt 2):870-6.
68. Lucas A, Morley R, Cole TJ, Gore SM. A randomised multicentre study of human milk versus formula and later development in preterm infants. *Arch Dis Child Fetal Neonatal Ed.* 1994;70(2):F141-6.
69. Rao MR, Hediger ML, Levine RJ, Naficy AB, Vik T. Effect of breastfeeding on cognitive development of infants born small for gestational age. *Acta Paediatr.* 2002;91(3):267-74.
70. Arnold LD. Global health policies that support the use of banked donor human milk: a human rights issue. *Int Breastfeed J.* 2006;1:26.
71. Poets CF, Langner MU, Bohnhorst B. Effects of bottle feeding and two different methods of gavage feeding on oxygenation and breathing patterns in preterm infants. *Acta Paediatr.* 1997;86:419-23.
72. Hamprecht K, Goelz R, Maschmann J. Breast milk and cytomegalovirus infection in preterm infants. *Early Hum Dev.* 2005;81:989-96.
73. Mehler K, Oberthuer A, Lang-Roth R, Kribs A. High rate of symptomatic cytomegalovirus infection in extremely low gestational age preterm infants of 22-24 weeks' gestation after transmission via breast milk. *Neonatology.* 2014;105:27-32.
74. Forsgren M. Cytomegalovirus in breast milk: reassessment of pasteurization and freeze-thawing. *Pediatr Res.* 2004;56:526-8.
75. Eglash A. ABM clinical protocol #8: human milk storage information for home use for full-term infants (original protocol March 2004; revision #1 March 2010). *Breastfeed Med.* 2010;5(3):127-30.
76. Boo NY, Nordiah AJ, Alfizah H, Nor-Rohaini AH, Lim VK. Contamination of breast milk obtained by manual expression and breast pumps in mothers of very low birthweight infants. *J Hosp Infect.* 2001;49(4):274-81.
77. Ng DK, Lee SYR, Leung LCK, Wong SF, Ho JCS. Bacteriological screening of expressed breast milk revealed a high rate of bacterial contamination in Chinese women. *J Hosp Infect.* 2004;58:146-50.
78. Dahaban NM, Romli MF, Roslan NR, Kong SS, Cheah FC. Bacteria in expressed breastmilk from mothers of premature infants and maternal hygienic status. *Breastfeed Med.* 2013;8(4):422-3.
79. Ewaschuk JB, Unger S, Harvey S, O'Connor DL, Field CJ. Effect of pasteurization on immune components of milk: implications for feeding preterm infants. *Appl Physiol Nutr Metab.* 2011;36:175-82.
80. Ahmed AH. Role of the pediatric nurse practitioner in promoting breastfeeding for late preterm infants in primary care settings. *J Pediatr Health Care.* 2010;24(2):116-22.
81. Black A. Breastfeeding the premature infant and nursing implications. *Adv Neonatal Care.* 2012;12:10-1.
82. Spatz DL. Ten steps for promoting and protecting breastfeeding for vulnerable infants. *J Perinat Neonatal Nurs.* 2004;18(4):385-96.

83. Prieto CR, Cardenas H, Salvatierra AM, Boza C, Montes CG, Croxatto HB. Sucking pressure and its relationship to milk transfer during breastfeeding in humans. *J Reprod Fertil.* 1996;108(1):69-74.
84. Mangel L, Ovental A, Batscha N, Arnon M, Yarkoni I, Dollberg S. Higher fat content in breast milk expressed manually: a randomised trial. *Breastfeed Med.* 2015;10(7):352-354.
85. Kent JC, Ramsay DT, Doherty D, Larsson M, Hartmann PE. Response of Breasts to Different Stimulation Patterns of an Electric Breast Pump. *J Hum Lact.* 2003;19:179-86.
86. Neville MC, Keller R, Seacat J, Lûtes V, Neifert M, Casey C, et al. Studies in human lactation: milk volumes in lactating women during the onset of lactation and full lactation. *Am J Clin Nutr.* 1988;48(6):1375-86.
87. Forinash AB, Yancey AM, Barnes KN, Myles TD. The use of galactogogues in the breastfeeding mother. *Ann Pharmacother.* 2012;46:1392-404.
88. Donovan TJ, Buchanan K. Medications for increasing milk supply in mothers expressing breastmilk for their preterm hospitalised infants. *Cochrane Database Syst Rev.* 2012;3:CD 005544.
89. Hsu HT, Fong TV, Hassan NM, Wong HL, Rai JK, Khalid Z. Human milk donation is an alternative to human milk bank. *Breastfeed Med.* 2012;7(2):118-22.
90. Bertino E, Peila C, Giuliani F, Martano C, Cresi F, Di Nicola P, et al. Metabolism and biological functions of human milk oligosaccharides. *J Biol Regul Homeost Agents.* 2012;26(3 Suppl):35-8.
91. Bode L. Human milk oligosaccharides: every baby needs a sugar mama. *Glycobiology.* 2012;22(9):1147-62.
92. Kunz C, Rudloff S, Baier W, Klein N, Strobel S. Oligosaccharides in human milk: structural, functional, and metabolic aspects. *Annu Rev Nutr.* 2000;20:699-722.
93. Urashima T, Saito T, Nakamura T, Messer M. Oligosaccharides of milk and colostrum in non-human mammals. *Glycoconj J.* 2001;18(5):357-71.
94. Kuschel CA, Harding JE. Protein supplementation of human milk for promoting growth in preterm infants. *Cochrane Database Syst Rev.* 2000(2):CD000433.
95. Perrine CG, Sharma AJ, Jefferds ME, Serdula MK, Scanlon KS. Adherence to vitamin D recommendations among US infants. *Pediatrics.* 2010;125(4):627-32.
96. Buyukuslu N, Esin K, Hizli H, Sunal N, Yigiy P, Garipagaoglu M. Clothing preference affects vitamin D status of young women. *Nut Res.* 2014;34(8):688-693.
97. Engelsen O. The relationship between ultraviolet radiation exposure and vitamin D status. *Nutrients.* 2010;2:482-495.
98. Demarini S. Calcium and phosphorus nutrition in preterm infants. *Acta Paediatr Suppl.* 2005;94(449):87-92.
99. Makrides M, Gibson RA, McPhee AJ, Collins CT, Davis PG, Doyle LW, et al. Neurodevelopmental outcomes of preterm infants fed high-dose docosahexaenoic acid: a randomized controlled trial. *JAMA.* 2009;301:175-82.
100. Manley BJ, Makrides M, Collins CT, McPhee AJ, Gibson RA, Ryan P, et al. High-dose docosahexaenoic acid supplementation of preterm infants: respiratory and allergy outcomes. *Pediatrics.* 2011;128:e71-7.
101. Saarela T, Kokkonen J, Koivisto M. Macronutrient and energy contents of human milk fractions during the first six months of lactation. *Acta Paediatr.* 2005;94:1176-81.
102. Weber A, Loui A, Jochum F, Buhrer C, Obladen M. Breast milk from mothers of very low birthweight infants: variability in fat and protein content. *Acta Paediatr.* 2001;90(7):772-5.
103. Cheah FC, Yiaw KW, Subramaniam B, Rasabar S, Mazwin N, Isa M. Monitoring the caloric content of breast milk by creamatocrit at the bedside: optimizing nutrient delivery for better growth of the preterm infant. *J Perinatal Med.* 2013;41.DOI 10.1515/jpm-2013-2003. (Abstract 665).
104. Cheah FC, Tiew WT, Raja Lope RJ, Ismail J. A randomised controlled trial comparing the effects of individualised and stardised fortification of expressed breast milk on the growth of preterm infants in the NICU. *J. Perinal Med.* 2015;43. Oral presentation no.:O-0242.

105. Arslanoglu S, Moro GE, Ziegler EE, The Wapm Working Group On N. Optimization of human milk fortification for preterm infants: new concepts and recommendations. *J Perinat Med.* 2010; 38(3):233-8.
106. Adamkin DH. Feeding the preterm infant. In Bhatia J (ed.). Perinatal nutrition: optimizing infant health and development. New York: Marcel Dekker 2005: pp 165-90.
107. Embleton NE, Pang N, Cooke RJ. Postnatal malnutrition and growth retardation: an inevitable consequence of current recommendations in preterm infants? *Pediatrics.* 2001;107(2):270-3.
108. Cooke RJ, Ainsworth SB, Fenton AC. Postnatal growth retardation: a universal problem in preterm infants. *Arch Dis Child Fetal Neonatal Ed.* 2004;89(5):F428-30.
109. Fanaroff AA, Stoll BJ, Wright LL, Carlo WA, Ehrenkranz RA, Stark AR, et al. Trends in neonatal morbidity and mortality for very low birthweight infants. *Am J Obstet Gynecol.* 2007;196(2):147 e1-8.
110. Henriksen C, Westerberg AC, Ronnestad A, Nakstad B, Veierod MB, Drevon CA, et al. Growth and nutrient intake among very-low-birth-weight infants fed fortified human milk during hospitalisation. *Br J Nutr.* 2009;102(8):1179-86.
111. Brandt I, Sticker EJ, Lentze MJ. Catch-up growth of head circumference of very low birth weight, small for gestational age preterm infants and mental development to adulthood. *J Pediatr.* 2003; 142(5):463-8.
112. Latal-Hajnal B, von Siebenthal K, Kovari H, Bucher HU, Largo RH. Postnatal growth in VLBW infants: significant association with neurodevelopmental outcome. *J Pediatr.* 2003;143(2):163-70.
113. Ehrenkranz RA, Dusick AM, Vohr BR, Wright LL, Wrage LA, Poole WK. Growth in the neonatal intensive care unit influences neurodevelopmental and growth outcomes of extremely low birth weight infants. *Pediatrics.* 2006;117(4):1253-61.
114. Ehrenkranz RA, Das A, Wrage LA, Poindexter BB, Higgins RD, Stoll BJ, et al. Early nutrition mediates the influence of severity of illness on extremely LBW infants. *Pediatr Res.* 2011;69(6):522-9.
115. Wilson DC, Cairns P, Halliday HL, Reid M, McClure G, Dodge JA. Randomised controlled trial of an aggressive nutritional regimen in sick very low birthweight infants. *Arch Dis Child Fetal Neonatal Ed.* 1997;77(1):F4-11.
116. Horbar JD, Badger GJ, Carpenter JH, Fanaroff AA, Kilpatrick S, LaCorte M, et al. Trends in mortality and morbidity for very low birth weight infants, 1991-1999. *Pediatrics.* 2002;110(1 Pt 1):143-51.
117. Kusuda S, Fujimura M, Sakuma I, Aotani H, Kabe K, Itani Y, et al. Morbidity and mortality of infants with very low birth weight in Japan: center variation. *Pediatrics.* 2006;118(4):e1130-8.
118. Barker DJ, Winter PD, Osmond C, Margetts B, Simmonds SJ. Weight in infancy and death from ischaemic heart disease. *Lancet.* 1989;2(8663):577-80.
119. Lucas A. Long-term programming effects of early nutrition -- implications for the preterm infant. *J Perinatol.* 2005;25 Suppl 2:S2-6.
120. Regan FM, Cutfield WS, Jefferies C, Robinson E, Hofman PL. The impact of early nutrition in premature infants on later childhood insulin sensitivity and growth. *Pediatrics.* 2006;118(5):1943-9.
121. Bertino E, Coscia A, Mombro M, Boni L, Rossetti G, Fabris C, et al. Postnatal weight increase and growth velocity of very low birthweight infants. *Arch Dis Child Fetal Neonatal Ed.* 2006;91 (5):F349-56.
122. National Healthcare Group Polyclinics anthropometric growth charts for pre-school children in Singapore 2000.
123. Lee PA, Chernausek SD, Hokken-Koelega AC, Czernichow P. International Small for Gestational Age Advisory Board consensus development conference statement: management of short children born small for gestational age, April 24-October 1, 2001. *Pediatrics.* 2003;111(6 Pt 1):1253-61.
124. Wojcik KY, Rechtman DJ, Lee ML, Montoya A, Medo ET. Macronutrient analysis of a nationwide sample of donor breast milk. *J Am Diet Assoc.* 2009;109(1):137-40.

125. Zachariassen G, Fenger-Gron J, Hviid MV, Halken S. The content of macronutrients in milk from mothers of very preterm infants is highly variable. Dan Med J. 2013;60(6):A4631.
126. Kuschel CA, Harding JE. Multicomponent fortified human milk for promoting growth in preterm infants. Cochrane Database Syst Rev. 2004(1):CD000343.
127. Sullivan S, Schanler RJ, Kim JH, Patel AL, Trawoger R, Kiechl-Kohlendorfer U, et al. An exclusively human milk-based diet is associated with a lower rate of necrotizing enterocolitis than a diet of human milk and bovine milk-based products. J Pediatr. 2010;156(4):562-7 e1.
128. Martin I, Jackson L. Question 1. Is there an increased risk of necrotising enterocolitis in preterm infants whose mothers' expressed breast milk is fortified with multicomponent fortifier? Arch Dis Child. 2011;96(12):1199-201.
129. Sauer CW, Kim JH. Human milk macronutrient analysis using point-of-care near-infrared spectrophotometry. J Perinatol. 2011;31(5):339-43.
130. Thakkar SK, Giuffrida F, Cristina CH, De Castro CA, Mukherjee R, Tran LA, et al. Dynamics of human milk nutrient composition of women from Singapore with a special focus on lipids. Am J Hum Biol. 2013;25(6):770-9.
131. Moya F, Sisk PM, Walsh KR, Berseth CL. A new liquid human milk fortifier and linear growth in preterm infants. Pediatrics. 2012;130(4):e928-35.
132. Miller J, Makrides M, Gibson RA, McPhee AJ, Stanford TE, Morris S, et al. Effect of increasing protein content of human milk fortifier on growth in preterm infants born at <31 wk gestation: a randomized controlled trial. Am J Clin Nutr. 2012;95(3):648-55.
133. Quigley M, McGuire W. Formula versus donor breast milk for feeding preterm or low birth weight infants. Cochrane Database Syst Rev. 2014;4:CD002971.
134. Boyd CA, Quigley MA, Brocklehurst P. Donor breast milk versus infant formula for preterm infants: systemic review and meta-analysis. Arch Dis Child Fetal Neonatol Ed. 2007;92:F169-175.
135. Horbar JD, Carpenter JH, Badger GJ, Kenny MJ, Soll RF, Morrow KA, et al. Mortality and neonatal morbidity among infants 501 to 1500 grams from 2000 to 2009. Pediatrics. 2012;129(6):1019-26.
136. Kamitsuka MD, Horton MK, Williams MA. The incidence of necrotizing enterocolitis after introducing standardized feeding schedules for infants between 1250 and 2500 grams and less than 35 weeks of gestation. Pediatrics. 2000;105(2):379-84.
137. Zhang SH, Yip WK, Lim PF, Goh MZ. Evidence utilization project: implementation of kangaroo care at neonatal ICU. Int J Evid Based Healthc. 2014;12(2):142-50.
138. Elgellab A, Riou Y, Abbazine A, Truffert P, Matran R, Lequien P, et al. Effects of nasal continuous positive airway pressure (NCPAP) on breathing pattern in spontaneously breathing premature newborn infants. Intensive Care Med. 2001;27(11):1782-7.
139. Miller M, Vaidya R, Rastogi D, Bhutada A, Rastogi S. From parenteral to enteral nutrition: a nutrition-based approach for evaluating postnatal growth failure in preterm infants. JPEN J Parenter Enteral Nutr. 2014;38(4):489-97.
140. Aggett PJ, Agostoni C, Axelsson I, De Curtis M, Goulet O, Hernell O, et al. Feeding preterm infants after hospital discharge: a commentary by the ESPGHAN Committee on Nutrition. J Pediatr Gastroenterol Nutr. 2006;42(5):596-603.
141. Katz J, Lee AC, Kozuki N, Lawn JE, Cousens S, Blencowe H, et al. Mortality risk in preterm and small-for-gestational-age infants in low-income and middle-income countries: a pooled country analysis. Lancet. 2013;382(9890):417-25.
142. Lee W, Balasubramaniam M, Deter RL et al. Fetal growth parameters and birth weight: their relationship to neonatal body composition. Ultrasound Obstet Gynecol. 2009;33(4):441-446.
143. Wen SW, Kramer MS, Usher RH. Comparison of birth weight distributions between Chinese and Caucasian infants. Am J Epidemiol. 1995;141:1177-87.

144. Janssen PA, Thiessen P, Klein MC, Whitfield MF, Macnab YC, Cullis-Kuhl SC. Standards for the measurement of birth weight, length and head circumference at term in neonates of European, Chinese and South Asian ancestry. *Open Med.* 2007;1:e74-88.

145. Harding S, Rosato MG, Cruickshank JK. Lack of change in birthweights of infants by generational status among Indian, Pakistani, Bangladeshi, Black Caribbean, and Black African mothers in a British cohort study. *Int J Epidemiol.* 2004;33:1279-85.

146. Lee ACC, Katz J, Blencowe H, Cousens S, Kozuki N, Vogel JP, et al. National and regional estimates of term and preterm babies born small for gestational age in 138 low-income and middle-income countries in 2010. *The Lancet Global Health.* 2013;1(1):e26-e36.

147. Dorling J, Kempley S, Leaf a. Feeding growth restricted preterm infants with abnormal antenatal Doppler results. *Arch Dis Child Fetal Neonatal Ed.* 2005;90:F359-63.

148. Kamoji VM, Dorling JS, Manktelow B, Draper ES, Field DJ. Antenatal umbilical Doppler abnormalities: an independent risk factor for early onset neonatal necrotizing enterocolitis in premature infants. *Acta Paediatr.* 2008;97:327-31.

149. Bora R, Mukhopadhyay K, Saxena AK, Jain V, Narang A. Prediction of feed intolerance and necrotizing enterocolitis in neonates with absent end diastolic flow in umbilical artery and the correlation of feed intolerance with postnatal superior mesenteric artery flow. *J Matern Fetal Neonatal Med.* 2009;22(11):1092-6.

150. Bozzetti V, Paterlini G, DeLorenzo P, Meroni V, Gazzolo D, Van Bel F, et al. Feeding tolerance of preterm infants appropriate for gestational age (AGA) as compared to those small for gestational age (SGA). *J Matern Fetal Neonatal Med.* 2013;26:1610-5.

151. Balion C, Grey V, Ismaila A, Blatz S, Seidlitz W. Screening for hypoglycemia at the bedside in the neonatal intensive care unit (NICU) with the Abbott PCx glucose meter. *BMC Pediatr.* 2006;6:28.

152. Beardsall K, Vanhaesebrouck S, Ogilvy-Stuart AL, Vanhole C, Palmer CR, Ong K, et al. Prevalence and determinants of hyperglycemia in very low birth weight infants: cohort analyses of the NIRTURE study. *J Pediatr.* 2010;157(5):715-9 e1-3.

153. Zecca E, Costa S, Barone G, Giordano L, Zecca C, Maggio L. Proactive enteral nutrition in moderately preterm small for gestational age infants: a randomized clinical trial. *J Pediatr.* 2014;165(6):1135-9 e1.

154. Kempley S, Gupta N, Linsell L, Dorling J, McCormick K, Mannix P, et al. Feeding infants below 29 weeks' gestation with abnormal antenatal Doppler: analysis from a randomised trial. *Arch Dis Child Fetal Neonatal Ed.* 2014;99:F6-F11.

155. Singhal A, Cole TJ, Fewtrell M, Kennedy K, Stephenson T, Elias-Jones A, et al. Promotion of faster weight gain in infants born small for gestational age: is there an adverse effect on later blood pressure? *Circulation.* 2007;115(2):213-20.

156. Hwa V, IGF-I in human growth: lessons from defects in the GH-IGF-I axis. *Nestle Nutr Inst Workshop Ser.* 2013;71:43-55.

157. Mussavi M, Asadollahi K, Abangah G. Effects of Metoclopramide on Feeding Intolerance among Preterm Neonates; A Randomized Controlled Trial. *Iran J Pediatr.* 2014;24(5):630-6.

158. Ng E, Shah VS. Erythromycin for the prevention and treatment of feeding intolerance in preterm infants. *Cochrane Database Syst Rev.* 2008(3):CD001815.

159. Aly H, Abdel-Hady H, Khashaba M, El-Badry N. Erythromycin and feeding intolerance in premature infants: a randomised trial. *Journal of Perinatology.* 2007;27:39-43.

160. Sices L, Wilson-Costello D, Minich N, Friedman H, Hack M. Postdischarge growth failure among extremely low birth weight infants: Correlates and consequences. *Paediatr Child Health.* 2007;12(1):22-8.

161. Goel KM, Gupta DK. Nutrition. In: Hutchinson's Paediatrics. Jaypee Brothers Medical Publishers Pvt. Ltd.,15 Dec 2012.

162. Ehrenkranz RA, Younes N, Lemons JA, Fanaroff AA, Donovan EF, Wright LL, et al. Longitudinal growth of hospitalized very low birth weight infants. *Pediatrics.* 1999;104:280-9.

163. Cooke RJ. Postdischarge nutrition of preterm infants: more questions than answers. *Nestlé Nutrition workshop series Paediatric programme.* 2007;59:213-27; discussion 24-8.
164. Cooke R. Nutrition of preterm infants after discharge. *Ann Nutr Metab.* 2011;58(Suppl 1): 32-36.
165. Lucas A et al. Randomised trial of nutrient enriched formula vs standard formula for postdischarge preterm infants. *Paediatrics.* 2001;108(3).
166. Rigo J, De Curtis M, Pieltain C, Picaud JC, Salle BL, Senterre J. Bone mineral metabolism in the micropremie. *Clin Perinatol.* 2000;27:147-70.
167. Goel KM, Gupta DK .What is catch-up growth and what is accelerated growth? In: Hutchinson's Paediatrics. Jaypee Brothers Medical Publishers Pvt. Ltd., 15 Dec 2012
168. Morley R, Fewtrell MS, Abbott RA, Stephenson T, MacFadyen U, Lucas A. Neurodevelopment in children born small for gestational age: a randomized trial of nutrient-enriched versus standard formula and comparison with a reference breastfed group. *Pediatrics.* 2004;113:515-21.
169. Tomashek KM, Shapiro-Mendoza CK, Weiss J, Kotelchuck M, Barfield W, Evans S, et al. Early discharge among late preterm and term newborns and risk of neonatal morbidity. *Semin Perinatol.* 2006;30:61-8.
170. Schulze KF, Stefanski M, Masterson J, Spinnazola R, Ramakrishnan R, Dell RB, et al. Energy expenditure, energy balance, and composition of weight gain in low birth weight infants fed diets of different protein and energy content. *J Pediatr.* 1987;110:753-9.
171. Cooke RJ, Griffin IJ, McCormick K. Adiposity is not altered in preterm infants fed with a nutrient-enriched formula after hospital discharge. *Pediatr Res.* 2010;67(6):660-4.
172. Agostoni C. Small-for-gestational-age infants need dietary quality more than quantity for their development: the role of human milk. *Acta Paediatr.* 2005;94:827-9.
173. Joint FAO-WHO Working Group Report on Drafting Guidelines for the Evaluation of Probiotics in Food 2012. Available at ftp://ftp.fao.org/es/esn/food/wgreport2.pdf (Accessed November 2015).
174. Lin PW, Stoll BJ. Necrotising enterocolitis. *Lancet.* 2006;368(9543):1271-83.
175. Henry MC, Moss RL. Neonatal necrotizing enterocolitis. *Semin Pediatr Surg.* 2008;17(2):98-109.
176. Hsueh W, Caplan MS, Qu XW, Tan XD, De Plaen IG, Gonzalez-Crussi F. Neonatal necrotizing enterocolitis: clinical considerations and pathogenetic concepts. *Pediatr Dev Pathol.* 2002;6(1):6-23.
177. Claud EC, Walker WA. Bacterial colonization, probiotics, and necrotizing enterocolitis. *J Clin Gastroenterol.* 2008;42 Suppl 2:S46-52.
178. Lin PW, Nasr TR, Stoll BJ. Necrotising enterocolitis: recent scientific advances in pathophysiology and prevention. *Semin Perinatol.* 2008;32:70-82.
179. Australian and New Zealand Neonatal Network. 2013 Report of the Australian and New Zealand Neonatal Network.2015.
180. Cotten CM, Oh W, McDonald S, Carlo W, Fanaroff AA, Duara S, et al. Prolonged hospital stay for extremely premature infants: risk factors, center differences, and the impact of mortality on selecting a best-performing center. *J Perinatol.* 2005;25(10):650-5.
181. Wales PW, Christison-Lagay ER. Short bowel syndrome: epidemiology and etiology. *Semin Pediatr Surg.* 2010;19(1):3-9.
182. Salvia G, Guarino A, Terrin G, Cascioli C, Paludetto R, Indrio F, et al. Neonatal onset intestinal failure: an Italian Multicenter Study. *J Pediatr.* 2008;153(5):674-6, 6 e1-2.
183. Schulzke SM, Deshpande GC, Patole SK. Neurodevelopmental outcomes of very low-birth-weight infants with necrotizing enterocolitis: a systematic review of observational studies. *Arch Pediatr Adolesc Med.* 2007;161(6):583-90.
184. Hintz SR, Kendrick DE, Stoll BJ, Vohr BR, Fanaroff AA, Donovan EF, et al. Neurodevelopmental and growth outcomes of extremely low birth weight infants after necrotizing enterocolitis. *Pediatrics.* 2005;115(3):696-703.

185. Bisquera JA, Cooper TR, Berseth CL. Impact of necrotizing enterocolitis on length of stay and hospital charges in very low birth weight infants. *Pediatrics.* 2002;109(3):423-8.
186. Athalye-Jape G, More K, Patole S. Progress in the field of necrotising enterocolitis--year 2012. *J Matern Fetal Neonatal Med.* 2013;26(7):625-32.
187. Martin CR, Walker WA. Probiotics: role in pathophysiology and prevention in necrotizing enterocolitis. *Semin Perinatol.* 2008;32(2):127-37.
188. Lawton EM, Ross RP, Hill C, Cotter PD. Two-peptide lantibiotics: a medical perspective. *Mini Rev Med Chem.* 2007;7(12):1236-47.
189. Rakoff-Nahoum S, Paglino J, Eslami-Varzaneh F, Edberg S, Medzhitov R. Recognition of commensal microflora by toll-like receptors is required for intestinal homeostasis. *Cell.* 2004;118(2):229-41.
190. Ewaschuk JB, Backer JL, Churchill TA, Obermeier F, Krause DO, Madsen KL. Surface expression of Toll-like receptor 9 is upregulated on intestinal epithelial cells in response to pathogenic bacterial DNA. *Infect Immun.* 2007;75(5):2572-9.
191. Veckman V, Miettinen M, Pirhonen J, Siren J, Matikainen S, Julkunen I. Streptococcus pyogenes and Lactobacillus rhamnosus differentially induce maturation and production of Th1-type cytokines and chemokines in human monocyte-derived dendritic cells. *J Leukoc Biol.* 2004;75(5):764-71.
192. Khailova L, Dvorak K, Arganbright KM, Halpern MD, Kinouchi T, Yajima M, et al. Bifidobacterium bifidum improves intestinal integrity in a rat model of necrotizing enterocolitis. *Am J Physiol Gastrointest Liver Physiol.* 2009;297(5):G940-9.
193. Liu Y, Fatheree NY, Mangalat N, Rhoads JM. Human-derived probiotic Lactobacillus reuteri strains differentially reduce intestinal inflammation. *Am J Physiol Gastrointest Liver Physiol.* 2010; 299(5):G1087-96.
194. Taupin D, Podolsky DK. Trefoil factors: initiators of mucosal healing. *Nat Rev Mol Cell Biol.* 2003;4(9):721-32.
195. Salzman NH, Underwood MA, Bevins CL. Paneth cells, defensins, and the commensal microbiota: a hypothesis on intimate interplay at the intestinal mucosa. *Semin Immunol.* 2007;19(2):70-83.
196. Bevins CL, Salzman NH. Paneth cells, antimicrobial peptides and maintenance of intestinal homeostasis. *Nat Rev Microbiol.* 2011;9(5):356-68.
197. Underwood MA, Kananurak A, Coursodon CF, Adkins-Reick CK, Chu H, Bennett SH, et al. Bifidobacterium bifidum in a rat model of necrotizing enterocolitis: antimicrobial peptide and protein responses. *Pediatr Res.* 2012;71(5):546-51.
198. Deshpande G, Rao S, Patole S. Probiotics for prevention of necrotising enterocolitis in preterm neonates with very low birthweight: a systematic review of randomised controlled trials. *Lancet.* 2007;369(9573):1614-20.
199. Deshpande G, Rao S, Patole S, Bulsara M. Updated meta-analysis of probiotics for preventing necrotizing enterocolitis in preterm neonates. *Pediatrics.* 2010;125(5):921-30.
200. AlFaleh K, Anabrees J. Probiotics for prevention of necrotizing enterocolitis in preterm infants. *Cochrane Database Syst Rev.* 2014;4:CD005496.
201. Jacobs SE, Tobin JM, Opie GF, Donath S, Tabrizi SN, Pirotta M, et al. Probiotic effects on late-onset sepsis in very preterm infants: a randomized controlled trial. *Pediatrics.* 2013;132(6):1055-62.
202. Athalye-Jape G, Deshpande G, Rao S, Patole S. Benefits of probiotics on enteral nutrition in preterm neonates: a systematic review. *Am J Clin Nutr.* 2014;100(6):1508-19.
203. Indrio F, Riezzo G, Raimondi F, Bisceglia M, Filannino A, Cavallo L, et al. Lactobacillus reuteri accelerates gastric emptying and improves regurgitation in infants. *Eur J Clin Invest.* 2011;41(4):417-22.
204. Indrio F, Riezzo G, Raimondi F, Bisceglia M, Cavallo L, Francavilla R. Effects of probiotic and prebiotic on gastrointestinal motility in newborns. *J Physiol Pharmacol.* 2009;60 Suppl 6:27-31.
205. Indrio F, Riezzo G, Raimondi F, Bisceglia M, Cavallo L, Francavilla R. The effects of probiotics on feeding tolerance, bowel habits, and gastrointestinal motility in preterm newborns. *J Pediatr.* 2008;152(6):801-6.

206. Liu Y, Tran DQ, Fatheree NY, Marc Rhoads J. Lactobacillus reuteri DSM 17938 differentially modulates effector memory T cells and Foxp3+ regulatory T cells in a mouse model of necrotizing enterocolitis. *Am J Physiol Gastrointest Liver Physiol.* 2014;307(2):G177-86.

207. Liu Y, Fatheree NY, Mangalat N, Rhoads JM. Lactobacillus reuteri strains reduce incidence and severity of experimental necrotizing enterocolitis via modulation of TLR4 and NF-kappaB signaling in the intestine. *Am J Physiol Gastrointest Liver Physiol.* 2012;302(6):G608-17.

208. Rosander A, Connolly E, Roos S. Removal of antibiotic resistance gene-carrying plasmids from Lactobacillus reuteri ATCC 55730 and characterization of the resulting daughter strain, L. reuteri DSM 17938. *Appl Environ Microbiol.* 2008;74(19):6032-40.

209. Hoyos AB. Reduced incidence of necrotizing enterocolitis associated with enteral administration of Lactobacillus acidophilus and Bifidobacterium infantis to neonates in an intensive care unit. *Int J Infect Dis.* 1999;3(4):197-202.

210. Satoh Y, Shinohara K, Umezaki H, Shoji H, Satoh H, Ohtsuka Y, Shiga S, Nagata S, Shimizu T, Yamashiro Y. Bifidobacteria prevents necrotising enterocolitis and infection. *Int J Probiot Prebiot.* 2007;2:149-54.

211. Manzoni P, Lista G, Gallo E, Marangione P, Priolo C, Fontana P, et al. Routine Lactobacillus rhamnosus GG administration in VLBW infants: a retrospective, 6-year cohort study. *Early Hum Dev.* 2011;87 Suppl 1:S35-8.

212. Luoto R, Isolauri E, Lehtonen L. Safety of Lactobacillus GG probiotic in infants with very low birth weight: twelve years of experience. *Clin Infect Dis.* 2010;50(9):1327-8.

213. Deshpande G, Shingde V, Downe L, Leroi M, Xiao J. Routine probiotics for preterm neonates: Experience in a tertiary Australian neonatal intensive care unit. Presented at European Academy of Pediatric Congress and Master course, September 17-20, 2015, Oslo, Norway. Abstract: EAP-1021-766

214. Janvier A, Malo J, Barrington KJ. Cohort study of probiotics in a North American neonatal intensive care unit. *J Pediatr.* 2014;164(5):980-5.

215. Hartel C, Pagel J, Rupp J, Bendiks M, Guthmann F, Rieger-Fackeldey E, et al. Prophylactic use of Lactobacillus acidophilus/Bifidobacterium infantis probiotics and outcome in very low birth weight infants. *J Pediatr.* 2014;165(2):285-9 e1.

216. Costeloe K, Hardy P, Juszczak E, Wilks M, Millar MR, Probiotics in Preterm Infants Study Collaborative Group. Bifidobacterium breve BBG-001 in very preterm infants: a randomised controlled phase 3 trial. *Lancet.* 2015;S0140-6736(15)01027-2. doi: 10.1016/S0140-6736(15)01027-2. [Epub ahead of print]

217. Enos MK, Burton JP, Dols J, Buhulata S, Changalucha J, Reid G. Probiotics and nutrients for the first 1000 days of life in the developing world. *Benef Microbes.* 2013;4(1):3-16.

218. Dutta S, Ray P, Narang A. Comparison of Stool Colonization in Premature Infants by Three Dose Regimes of a Probiotic Combination: A Randomized Controlled Trial. *Am J Perinatol.* 2015;32(8):733-40.

219. Awad H, Mokhtar H, Imam SS, Gad GI, Hafez H, Aboushady N. Comparison between killed and living probiotic usage versus placebo for the prevention of necrotizing enterocolitis and sepsis in neonates. *Pak J Biol Sci.* 2010;13:253-62.

220. Yang Y, Guo Y, Kan Q, Zhou XG, Zhou XY, Li Y. A meta-analysis of probiotics for preventing necrotizing enterocolitis in preterm neonates. *Braz J Med Biol Res.* 2014;47(9):804-10.

221. Bernardo WM, Aires FT, Carneiro RM, Sa FP, Rullo VE, Burns DA. Effectiveness of probiotics in the prophylaxis of necrotizing enterocolitis in preterm neonates: a systematic review and meta-analysis. *J Pediatr (Rio J).* 2013;89(1):18-24.

222. Wang Q, Dong J, Zhu Y. Probiotic supplement reduces risk of necrotizing enterocolitis and mortality in preterm very low-birth-weight infants: an updated meta-analysis of 20 randomized, controlled trials. *J Pediatr Surg.* 2012;47:241-8.

223. Oncel MY, Sari FN, Arayici S, Guzoglu N, Erdeve O, Uras N, et al. Lactobacillus Reuteri for the prevention of necrotising enterocolitis in very low birthweight infants: a randomised controlled trial. *Arch Dis Child Fetal Neonatal Ed.* 2014;99(2):F110-5.

224. Samanta M, Sarkar M, Ghosh P, Ghosh J, Sinha M, Chatterjee S. Prophylactic probiotics for prevention of necrotizing enterocolitis in very low birth weight newborns. *J Trop Pediatr.* 2009; 55(2):128-31.

225. Roy A, Chaudhuri J, Sarkar D, Ghosh P, Chakraborty S. Role of Enteric Supplementation of Probiotics on Late-onset Sepsis by Candida species in Preterm Low Birth Weight Neonates: A Randomized, Double Blind, Placebo-controlled Trial. *N Am J Med Sci.* 2014;6(1):50-7.

226. Musilova S, Rada V, Vlkova E, Bunesova V. Beneficial effects of human milk oligosaccharides on gut microbiota. *Benef Microbes.* 2014;5(3):273-83.

227. Turin CG, Ochoa TJ. The Role of Maternal Breast Milk in Preventing Infantile Diarrhea in the Developing World. *Curr Trop Med Rep.* 2014;1(2):97-105.

228. Ballard O, Morrow AL. Human milk composition: nutrients and bioactive factors. *Pediatr Clin North Am.* 2013;60(1):49-74.

229. Barile D, Rastall RA. Human milk and related oligosaccharides as prebiotics. *Curr Opin Biotechnol.* 2013;24(2):214-9.

230. Ruiz-Moyano S, Totten SM, Garrido DA, Smilowitz JT, German JB, Lebrilla CB, et al. Variation in consumption of human milk oligosaccharides by infant gut-associated strains of Bifidobacterium breve. *Appl Environ Microbiol.* 2013;79(19):6040-9.

231. Kunz C. Historical aspects of human milk oligosaccharides. *Adv Nutr.* 2012;3(3):430S-9S.

232. Rudloff S, Kunz C. Milk oligosaccharides and metabolism in infants. *Adv Nutr.* 2012;3(3):398S-405S.

233. Marcobal A, Sonnenburg JL. Human milk oligosaccharide consumption by intestinal microbiota. *Clin Microbiol Infect.* 2012;18 Suppl 4:12-5.

234. Marx C, Bridge R, Wolf AK, Rich W, Kim JH, Bode L. Human milk oligosaccharide composition differs between donor milk and mother's own milk in the NICU. *J Hum Lact.* 2014;30(1):54-61.

235. Hennet T, Weiss A, Borsig L. Decoding breast milk oligosaccharides. *Swiss Med Wkly.* 2014; 144:w13927.

236. Holscher HD, Davis SR, Tappenden KA. Human milk oligosaccharides influence maturation of human intestinal Caco-2Bbe and HT-29 cell lines. *J Nutr.* 2014;144(5):586-91.

237. Newburg DS. Glycobiology of human milk. *Biochemistry (Mosc).* 2013;78(7):771-85.

238. Ruhaak LR, Lebrilla CB. Analysis and role of oligosaccharides in milk. *BMB Rep.* 2012;45(8):442-51.

239. Bruzzese E, Volpicelli M, Squaglia M, Tartaglione A, Guarino A. Impact of prebiotics on human health. *Dig Liver Dis.* 2006;38 Suppl 2:S283-7.

240. Jeong K, Nguyen V, Kim J. Human milk oligosaccharides: the novel modulator of intestinal microbiota. *BMB Rep.* 2012;45(8):433-41.

241. Peterson R, Cheah WY, Grinyer J, Packer N. Glycoconjugates in human milk: protecting infants from disease. *Glycobiology.* 2013;23(12):1425-38.

242. Newburg DS. Neonatal protection by an innate immune system of human milk consisting of oligosaccharides and glycans. *J Anim Sci.* 2009;87(13 Suppl):26-34.

243. Kunz C, Rudloff S. Potential anti-inflammatory and anti-infectious effects of human milk oligosaccharides. *Adv Exp Med Biol.* 2008;606:455-65.

244. Jeurink PV, van Esch BC, Rijnierse A, Garssen J, Knippels LM. Mechanisms underlying immune effects of dietary oligosaccharides. *Am J Clin Nutr.* 2013;98(2):572S-7S.

245. Jantscher-Krenn E, Zherebtsov M, Nissan C, Goth K, Guner YS, Naidu N, et al. The human milk oligosaccharide disialyllacto-N-tetraose prevents necrotising enterocolitis in neonatal rats. *Gut.* 2012;61(10):1417-25.

246. Garrido D, Dallas DC, Mills DA. Consumption of human milk glycoconjugates by infant-associated bifidobacteria: mechanisms and implications. *Microbiology.* 2013;159(Pt 4):649-64.
247. Scholtens PA, Goossens DA, Staiano A. Stool characteristics of infants receiving short-chain galacto-oligosaccharides and long-chain fructo-oligosaccharides: a review. *World J Gastroenterol.* 2014;20(37):13446-52.
248. Oozeer R, van Limpt K, Ludwig T, Ben Amor K, Martin R, Wind RD, et al. Intestinal microbiology in early life: specific prebiotics can have similar functionalities as human-milk oligosaccharides. *Am J Clin Nutr.* 2013;98(2):561S-71S.
249. Yu ZT, Chen C, Newburg DS. Utilization of major fucosylated and sialylated human milk oligosaccharides by isolated human gut microbes. *Glycobiology.* 2013;23(11):1281-92.
250. Srinivasjois R, Rao S, Patole S. Prebiotic supplementation in preterm neonates: updated systematic review and meta-analysis of randomised controlled trials. *Clin Nutr.* 2013;32(6):958-65.
251. Niele N, van Zwol A, Westerbeek EA, Lafeber HN, van Elburg RM. Effect of non-human neutral and acidic oligosaccharides on allergic and infectious diseases in preterm infants. *Eur J Pediatr.* 2013;172(3):317-23.
252. Rao S, Srinivasjois R, Patole S. Prebiotic supplementation in full-term neonates: a systematic review of randomized controlled trials. *Arch Pediatr Adolesc Med.* 2009;163(8):755-64.
253. Osborn DA, Sinn JK. Prebiotics in infants for prevention of allergy. *Cochrane Database Syst Rev.* 2013;3:CD006474.
254. Giovannini M, Verduci E, Gregori D, Ballali S, Soldi S, Ghisleni D, et al. Prebiotic effect of an infant formula supplemented with galacto-oligosaccharides: randomized multicenter trial. *J Am Coll Nutr.* 2014;33(5):385-93.
255. Partty A, Luoto R, Kalliomaki M, Salminen S, Isolauri E. Effects of early prebiotic and probiotic supplementation on development of gut microbiota and fussing and crying in preterm infants: a randomized, double-blind, placebo-controlled trial. *J Pediatr.* 2013;163(5):1272-7 e1-2.
256. Ganguli K, Walker WA. Probiotics in the prevention of necrotizing enterocolitis. *J Clin Gastroenterol.* 2011;45 Suppl:S133-8.
257. WHO, UNICEF, Welstart International. Baby-friendly hospital initiative : revised, updated and expanded for integrated care. Section 1, Background and implementation. 2009. Available at http://apps.who.int/iris/bitstream/10665/43593/1/9789241594967_eng.pdf. (Accessed September 2015)
258. Bagci Bosi AT, Eriksen KG, Sobko T, Wijnhoven TM, Breda J. Breastfeeding practices and policies in WHO European Region Member States. *Public Health Nutr.* 2015:1-12.
259. Flacking R, Nyqvist KH, Ewald U. Effects of socioeconomic status on breastfeeding duration in mothers of preterm and term infants. *Eur J Public Health.* 2007;17(6):579-84.
260. Statistics Indonesia (Badan Pusat Statistik—BPS), National Population and Family Planning Board (BKKBN), and Kementerian Kesehatan (Kemenkes—MOH), and ICF International. 2013. Indonesia Demographic and Health Survey 2012. Jakarta, Indonesia: BPS, BKKBN, Kemenkes, and ICF International.
261. Fatimah S, Jr., Siti Saadiah HN, Tahir A, Hussain Imam MI, Ahmad Faudzi Y. Breastfeeding in Malaysia: Results of the Third National Health and Morbidity Survey (NHMS III) 2006. *Malays J Nutr.* 2010;16(2):195-206.
262. National Institute of Population Research and Training (NIPORT), Mitra and Associates, and ICF International. 2015. Bangladesh Demographic and Health Survey 2014: Key Indicators. Dhaka, Bangladesh, and Rockville, Maryland, USA: NIPORT, Mitra and Associates, and ICF International.
263. National Institute of Population Studies (NIPS) [Pakistan] and ICF International. 2013. Pakistan Demographic and Health Survey 2012-13. Islamabad, Pakistan, and Calverton, Maryland, USA: NIPS and ICF International.
264. Chua L, Win AM. Prevalence of breastfeeding in Singapore. Statistics Singapore Newsletter. Singapore 2013. Available at www.singstat.gov.sg. (Accessed September 2015)

265. Tarrant M, Wu KM, Fong DY, Lee IL, Wong EM, Sham A, et al. Impact of baby-friendly hospital practices on breastfeeding in Hong Kong. *Birth*. 2011;38(3):238-45.

266. Wang W, Lau Y, Chow A, Chan KS. Breast-feeding intention, initiation and duration among Hong Kong Chinese women: a prospective longitudinal study. *Midwifery*. 2014;30(6):678-87.

267. Mathur NB, Dhingra D. Perceived breast milk insufficiency in mothers of neonates hospitalized in neonatal intensive care unit. *Indian J Pediatr*. 2009;76(10):1003-6.

268. Ho I, Holroyd E. Chinese women's perceptions of the effectiveness of antenatal education in the preparation for motherhood. *J Adv Nurs*. 2002;38(1):74-85.

269. Tahir NM, Al-Sadat N. Does telephone lactation counselling improve breastfeeding practices? A randomised controlled trial. *Int J Nurs Stud*. 2013;50(1):16-25.

270. Gunanegara RF, Suryawan A, Sastrawinata US, Surachman T. Efektivitas Ekstrak Daun Katuk dalam Produksi Air Susu Ibu untuk Keberhasilan Menyusui- Article in Indonesian. *JKM*. 2010; 9(2):104-117.

271. Tengku AT, Wan AM, Zaharah S, Rohana AJ, Nik Normanieza NM. Perceptions and practice of exclusive breastfeeding among Malay women in Kelantan, Malaysia: a qualitative approach. *Malays J Nutr*. 2012;18(1):15-25.

272. Hishamshah M, Ramzan M, Rashid A, Mustaffa WW, Haroon R, Badaruddin N. Belief and Practices of Traditional Post Partum Care Among a Rural Community in Penang Malaysia. *The Internet Journal of Third World Medicine*. 2010;9(2).http://ispub.com/IJTWM/9/2/4210.

273. Manderson L. 'These are modern times': infant feeding practice in Peninsular Malaysia. *Soc Sci Med*. 1984;18(1):47-57.

274. Dixon G. Colostrum avoidance and early infant feeding in Asian societies. *Asia Pac J Clin Nutr*. 1992;1(4):225-9.

275. Tan KL. Factors associated with exclusive breastfeeding among infants under six months of age in peninsular malaysia. *Int Breastfeed J*. 2011;6(1):2.

276. Amin RM, Said ZM, Sutan R, Shah SA, Darus A, Shamsuddin K. Work related determinants of breastfeeding discontinuation among employed mothers in Malaysia. *Int Breastfeed J*. 2011;6(1):4.

277. Tarrant M, Fong DY, Wu KM, Lee IL, Wong EM, Sham A, et al. Breastfeeding and weaning practices among Hong Kong mothers: a prospective study. *BMC Pregnancy Childbirth*. 2010;10:27.

278. Kushwaha KP, Sankar J, Sankar MJ, Gupta A, Dadhich JP, Gupta YP, et al. Effect of peer counselling by mother support groups on infant and young child feeding practices: the Lalitpur experience. *PLoS One*. 2014;9(11):e109181.

www.ingramcontent.com/pod-product-compliance
Lightning Source LLC
Chambersburg PA
CBHW021942170526
45157CB00003B/894